SUGAR DETOX DIET COOKBOOK FOR WOMEN

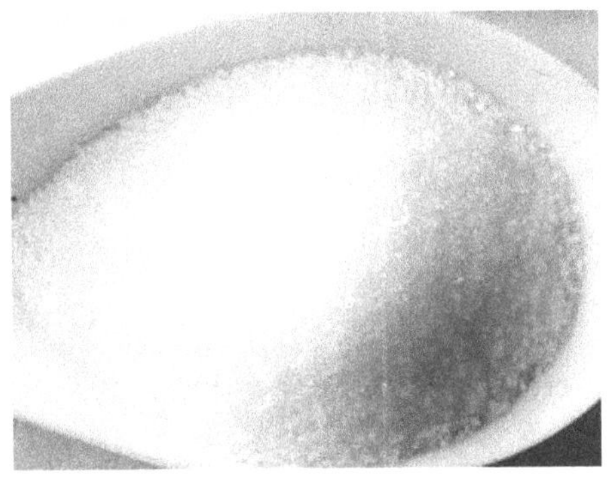

Delicious and simple recipes to lose weight for women

NAOMI PERCY

COPYRIGHT PAGE

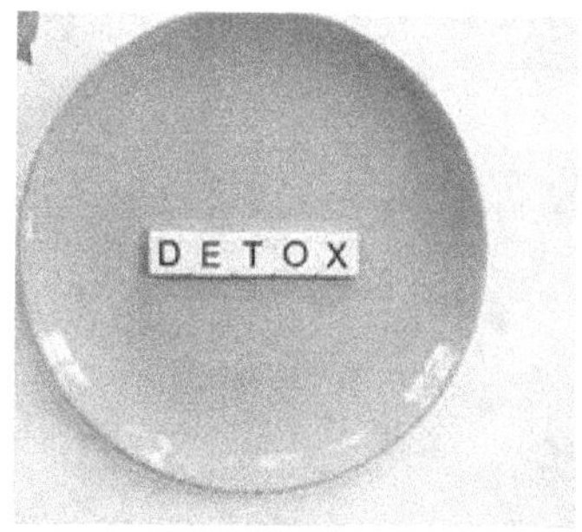

Table of Contents:

Introduction

As a woman who had struggled for years with sugar cravings and weight issues, my journey toward overcoming these challenges and achieving a healthier lifestyle began when I discovered the Sugar Detox recipes and made a 30-Day Plan for myself. It was a turning point that not only changed the way I ate but also transformed my entire life.

Like many others, I had a sweet tooth that seemed insatiable. I would reach for sugary snacks whenever I felt stressed or tired, thinking they were my source of comfort. But, over time, those moments of indulgence had taken a toll on my body. I had gained excess weight, felt sluggish, and my self-esteem had plummeted. I knew something had to change.

One day, while trying to fit into a dress for a party without much success I realized that my cravings for sugar and extremely sweet things is not good for my health so I have to do something about it and that's when I began my research on recipes that does not have sugar but give me delicious meals. And hence the beginning of my 30 days sugar detox plan. The plan worked so well and I was able to shed a good amount of calories and also make healthy and delicious meals and decided to combine the recipes together to help other women. This cookbook promised not only a way to break free from sugar's hold but also a path toward weight loss and overall wellness.

As I progressed through the weeks, I discovered a whole new world of delicious, sugar-free recipes. The breakfasts, lunches, dinners and smoothies were not only satisfying but also easy to prepare. I was amazed at how vibrant and flavorful food could be without added sugars.

What struck me the most during my sugar detox was how my cravings gradually diminished. The cookbook had helped me retrain my taste buds and my relationship with food. I was no longer a slave to sugar's seductive allure. Instead, I found satisfaction in the natural sweetness of fruits and vegetables.

By the end of the 30-day plan, I had not only shed those extra pounds that had been weighing me down for so long but had also gained a newfound sense of confidence and self-worth. I had more energy, my skin had cleared up, and I felt like a completely different person.

But the true beauty of this transformation was that it didn't end with the 30 days. The Sugar Detox Cookbook had equipped me with the knowledge and tools to make lasting changes in my life. I continued to enjoy the recipes and apply the principles I had learned, allowing me to maintain my weight loss and newfound vitality.

My journey with the Sugar Detox Cookbook and 30-Day Plan for Women wasn't just about losing weight; it was also about reclaiming my health, my self-esteem, and my love for wholesome, nourishing food. It showed me that with determination, the right guidance, and a commitment to change, I could overcome the hold that sugar had on me and embrace a healthier, happier future.

Welcome to the Sugar Detox Diet Cookbook for Women, your essential guide to begin on a transformative journey towards a healthier, slimmer and more vibrant you. In a world where sugar-laden temptations seem to lurk around every corner, this cookbook has been carefully crafted to empower you with the knowledge, recipes, and strategies needed to conquer sugar cravings, shed excess weight, and reclaim control over your health.

The influence of sugar on our lives is undeniable. It tantalizes our taste buds, provides momentary comfort, and even sneaks its way into foods we never suspected. However, beneath its sweet facade, sugar hides a darker side, one that can contribute to weight gain, low energy levels, and a host of health issues. For many women, it becomes a formidable obstacle on the path to achieving their ideal weight and overall wellness.

But fear not, for this cookbook is your ally in the battle against sugar. Within these pages, you will discover a carefully curated collection of recipes designed to not only help you break free from the grip of sugar but also delight your palate with an array of delicious, satisfying dishes. Whether you're starting your day with a nutritious breakfast, enjoying a hearty lunch, savoring a guilt-free dessert, or relaxing with a satisfying smoothie this recipes will prove that eating well can be both a pleasure and a path to progress.

But this cookbook is more than just a collection of recipes. It is a comprehensive resource that will guide you through the process of adopting a sugar detox diet tailored specifically for women. You'll learn how to assess your current sugar intake, set realistic weight loss goals, and create a shopping list that supports your newfound commitment to healthier eating. We'll also delve into the art of meal planning, a fundamental skill that will make your sugar detox journey smooth and sustainable.

Throughout this cookbook, you'll find chapters dedicated to various meals, snacks and smoothies, all carefully designed to keep you satisfied and energized while promoting weight loss. Our recipes use wholesome, nutrient-rich ingredients that not only support your goals but also make every meal a pleasure to prepare and enjoy.

As you begin this sugar detox adventure, we'll also provide guidance on managing sugar cravings, incorporating sugar into your diet mindfully, and ultimately, sustaining your newfound lifestyle. We believe that the Sugar Detox Diet Cookbook for Women will not only help you shed unwanted pounds but also empower you to make lasting changes for a lifetime of health and vitality.

So, turn the page, embrace the journey, and prepare to rediscover the joy of eating while achieving the weight loss and wellness goals you've always desired. Your sugar detox transformation begins here, and we are here to support you every step of the way.

In our modern world, sugar is everywhere. It's in the obvious places like candy and soda, but it also hides in seemingly innocent foods like cereal, yogurt, and even salad dressings. For women, the impact of sugar on our health can be profound, affecting everything from our weight to our overall well-being.

It's essential to grasp the role that sugar plays in our bodies and how it can influence our health as women. By doing so, we can make informed choices about our diets and embark on a journey toward better health and a more balanced lifestyle. Let's explore the key aspects of how sugar impacts your health:

Weight Gain: One of the most significant concerns for many women is weight management. Excessive sugar consumption can contribute to weight gain as it provides empty calories without significant nutritional value. Sugar triggers the release of insulin, a hormone that stores excess glucose as fat. This hormonal response can make it challenging to shed those unwanted pounds.

Energy Levels: While sugar can provide a quick energy boost, it's often followed by a crash. The rollercoaster of blood sugar spikes and crashes can leave you feeling tired and irritable. As a woman, maintaining steady energy levels is crucial for managing the demands of daily life.

Skin Health: Sugar can have a detrimental impact on your skin. Excess sugar intake has been the reason for some skin issues such as acne and premature aging. By reducing your sugar intake, you may notice improvements in your complexion and overall skin health.

Hormonal Balance: Sugar can disrupt hormonal balance in women, leading to irregular menstrual cycles and exacerbating symptoms of conditions like polycystic ovary syndrome (PCOS). Managing sugar consumption can contribute to more stable hormone levels.

 The sugar-insulin rollercoaster can also affect your mood. High sugar intake has been associated with mood swings, anxiety, and even depression. As women, maintaining emotional well-being is crucial, and understanding the link between sugar and mood can help you achieve that balance.

 Elevated sugar consumption is linked to heart disease, a leading cause of death among women. High sugar intake can raise blood pressure, increase bad cholesterol levels, and contribute to inflammation in the body, all of which are risk factors for heart disease.

 Excessive sugar intake can negatively impact your digestive system. It can disrupt the balance of beneficial bacteria in your gut and contribute to issues like bloating and constipation.

As you delve into the Sugar Detox Cookbook, remember that this journey is about more than just losing weight; it's about regaining control over your health and well-being as a woman. By understanding how sugar affects your body and embracing the sugar detox principles outlined in this cookbook, you're taking a significant step toward a healthier, happier, and more vibrant you.

The Benefits of a Sugar Detox

A sugar detox diet can be a transformative experience for women, offering a multitude of physical, emotional, and even psychological benefits. Breaking free from the shackles of excessive sugar consumption can lead to improved health, enhanced well-being, and a renewed sense

of vitality. Let's explore the many advantages that a sugar detox diet can bring to the lives of women:

Weight Management: Perhaps one of the most sought-after benefits for many women is weight loss. A sugar detox diet can help shed those stubborn pounds by reducing calorie intake and regulating insulin levels. Without the constant spikes and crashes in blood sugar that sugar consumption can trigger, maintaining a healthy weight becomes more achievable.

Stable Energy Levels: As busy women juggling multiple roles and responsibilities, having steady energy throughout the day is essential. A sugar detox diet can provide a sustained source of energy, preventing the energy crashes that often follow sugar consumption. This means improved focus, productivity, and overall vitality.

Enhanced Mood and Mental Clarity: Refined sugars and excessive carbohydrates can wreak havoc on mood stability. A sugar detox diet can help stabilize blood sugar levels, reducing mood swings, irritability, and even symptoms of anxiety and depression. Clearer thinking and improved mental clarity are additional perks.

Better Skin Health: Sugar is known to contribute to skin issues such as acne and premature aging. By reducing sugar intake, women often notice improvements in skin complexion, reduced blemishes, and a more youthful appearance.

Hormonal Balance: Hormonal imbalances can affect women's health in various ways, from irregular menstrual cycles to exacerbating conditions like polycystic ovary syndrome (PCOS). A sugar detox diet can help regulate hormones, potentially leading to more regular menstrual cycles and reduced PCOS symptoms.

Heart Health: Heart disease is a significant concern for women, and a sugar detox diet can be a powerful tool in preventing it. By reducing sugar intake, you can lower blood pressure, decrease levels of bad cholesterol, and reduce inflammation in the body, all of which are risk factors for heart disease.

Improved Digestive Health: Excessive sugar intake can disrupt the balance of beneficial gut bacteria, leading to digestive issues like bloating, gas, and constipation. A sugar detox diet can promote a healthier gut micro biome and alleviate these problems.

Reduced Risk of Chronic Diseases: Excessive sugar

consumption has been linked to a higher risk of chronic diseases such as type 2 diabetes and certain cancers. By detoxing from sugar, women can reduce their risk of these life-altering conditions and improve their overall health outlook.

Increased Longevity: A sugar detox diet can contribute to a longer, healthier life. By reducing the consumption of a substance known to contribute to various health problems, women can increase their chances of living a full, active life well into their later years.

Boosted Self-Esteem: Achieving and maintaining a healthier weight, clearer skin, and better overall health can significantly boost self-esteem and body confidence. Women who undergo a successful sugar detox often report feeling more confident and positive about themselves.

In summary, a sugar detox diet can provide a wealth of benefits for women, ranging from physical improvements in weight and skin health to emotional enhancements like mood stabilization and increased self-esteem. By embracing this journey toward reduced sugar consumption, women can take a proactive step toward achieving optimal health and well-being for the long term.

How This Cookbook and Plan Can Transform Your Life

Beginning a sugar detox journey through the pages of the Sugar Detox Cookbook for Women is about revamping your entire life, not just what you eat. This effective tool has the ability to transform your relationship with food, empower you to make better choices, and bring about a slew of beneficial changes that go well beyond the kitchen. Let's look at how this recipe and strategy may help you make a significant change in your life:

Improved Health: At its core, a sugar detox is about prioritizing your health. By reducing your sugar intake and embracing the wholesome, nutrient-rich recipes in this cookbook, you're taking a proactive step toward a healthier future. You'll likely experience weight loss, stabilized blood sugar levels, and reduced risk factors for chronic diseases, ultimately contributing to a longer, more vibrant life.

Enhanced Energy and Vitality: Say goodbye to the energy rollercoaster that sugar often creates. The carefully crafted recipes in this cookbook provide sustained energy throughout the day, allowing you to feel more alert, focused, and ready to tackle life's challenges with gusto.

Mood and Mental Clarity: The impact of sugar on mood stability is well-documented. By regulating your blood sugar levels through a sugar detox, you can experience fewer mood swings, reduced anxiety, and improved mental clarity. This newfound emotional balance can positively affect your relationships and overall quality of life.

Confidence and Self-Esteem: Achieving and maintaining a healthier weight and clearer skin can significantly boost self-esteem and body confidence. As you witness the positive changes in your appearance and feel more in control of your health, you'll carry yourself with newfound self-assuredness.

Guilt-Free Pleasure: The Sugar Detox Cookbook is a treasure trove of recipes that prove you don't have to sacrifice taste for health. These dishes are not just nourishing; they're delicious. You can savor each bite guilt-free, knowing that you're nourishing your body and satisfying your palate simultaneously.

Empowerment and Knowledge: Knowledge is power, and this cookbook equips you with valuable information about sugar, nutrition, and meal planning. Armed with this knowledge, you'll feel empowered to make informed choices about what you eat, setting you on a path to a lifetime of healthier eating habits.

Sustainable Lifestyle Change: The Sugar Detox Cookbook and 30-Day Plan is not a crash diet; it's a blueprint for lasting change. By following the principles outlined in this resource, you'll develop the skills and mindset needed to maintain a low-sugar, healthy lifestyle for years to come.

 The journey to a sugar-free lifestyle can be more enjoyable and successful when you have support. Whether it's sharing recipes with friends, participating in online communities, or involving loved ones in your journey, this cookbook can foster a sense of camaraderie that makes the transformation more manageable.

 A sugar detox isn't just about physical health; it's an opportunity for personal growth. It requires discipline, determination, and self-reflection. As you conquer sugar cravings and make healthier choices, you'll likely find yourself growing in resilience and self-awareness.

In conclusion, the Sugar Detox Cookbook for Women is more than a collection of recipes; it's a life-changing resource that has the potential to revolutionize the way you eat, think, and live. It offers the promise of improved health, elevated energy levels, heightened self-esteem, and a newfound sense of empowerment. Embrace this journey with an open heart and an appetite for transformation, and watch as it positively impacts every aspect of your life.

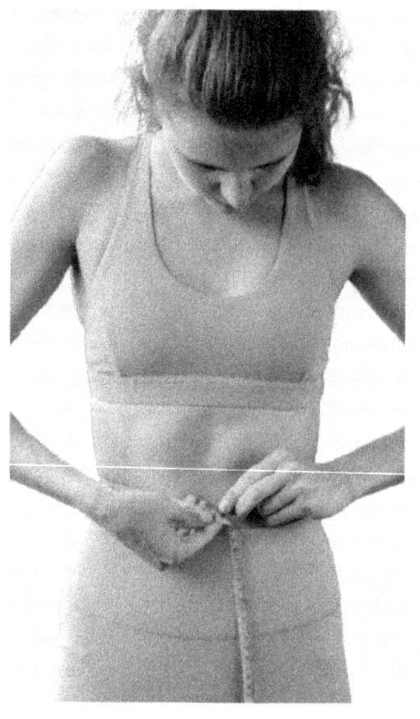

Chapter 1:

Preparing for Your Sugar Detox

Starting a sugar detox is a positive start toward better health and weight loss. It's a vow to break free from sugar's enticing grasp and reclaim control over your eating habits. Proper planning is essential for success during the first part of your sugar detox. Here's a detailed guide on preparing for your sugar detox:

1. Self-Assessment: Begin your sugar detox journey by taking stock of your current dietary habits. Keep a food diary for a few days to track your sugar consumption. This will help you understand your sugar triggers and identify areas where you need to make changes.

2. Set Clear Goals: Define your objectives for the sugar detox. Whether it's weight loss, improved energy levels, clearer skin, or better mood, having

clear and realistic goals will keep you motivated throughout the process.

3. Educate Yourself: **Knowledge is your best ally in this journey. Learn about the different types of sugars, where they hide in foods, and how to identify them on nutrition labels. This knowledge will give you the power to make informed choices.**

4. Clear Your Pantry: **Before starting your sugar detox, take the time to clean out your pantry, refrigerator, and kitchen cabinets. Remove all sugary and processed foods that may tempt you during your detox. Replace them with wholesome, sugar-free alternatives.**

5. Create a Shopping List: **Prepare a comprehensive shopping list that includes the fresh, whole foods you'll need for your detox. Focus on fruits, vegetables, lean proteins, whole grains, nuts, and seeds. Making these items ready and available will make it easier to maintain your detox plan.**

6. Meal Planning: **Plan your meals and snacks for the first week of your detox. Having a meal plan in**

place will prevent you from reaching for sugary snacks out of convenience. The Sugar Detox Cookbook for Women can be an excellent resource for recipe ideas and meal planning inspiration.

7. Hydration: Ensure you stay well-hydrated throughout your detox by drinking plenty of water. Hydration can help curb cravings and support the detoxification process.

8. Support System: Share your detox journey with friends or family who can offer encouragement and accountability. Having a support system can be instrumental in staying on track.

9. Mindset: Approach your sugar detox with a positive mindset. Instead of viewing it as a restrictive diet, see it as an opportunity to nourish your body and prioritize your health. Cultivate self-compassion and be patient with yourself during the process.

10. Alternatives: Explore sugar alternatives like stevia, monk fruit, or erythritol if you find it challenging to completely eliminate sweetness from

your diet. These can be used sparingly to satisfy your sweet tooth without derailing your detox.

11. Journaling: Consider keeping a journal to document your sugar detox journey. Note your thoughts, feelings, and physical changes throughout the process. It can be a valuable tool for self-reflection and motivation.

By taking these steps to prepare for your sugar detox, you're setting yourself up for a successful and transformative experience. Remember that a sugar detox is not just about eliminating sugar; it's about embracing a healthier, more mindful way of eating that can lead to lasting weight loss and improved well-being. Prepare diligently, stay committed to your goals, and get ready to reap the benefits of a sugar-free lifestyle.

Assessing Your Current Sugar Intake

Before diving headfirst into your sugar detox diet for women, it's essential to have a clear understanding of your current sugar consumption. This self-assessment will serve as a valuable baseline for measuring your progress throughout the detox and help you identify areas where sugar may be sneaking into your diet unnoticed. Here's how to assess your sugar intake effectively:

1. Keep a Food Diary: Start by keeping a detailed food diary for at least one week. Record everything you eat and drink, including portion sizes and any added sugars. Be meticulous in your documentation, noting even the seemingly insignificant sources of sugar, such as that teaspoon of sugar in your morning coffee or the condiments you use in your meals.

2. Read Labels: Pay close attention to food labels. Many processed foods, even those that don't taste sweet, contain added sugars. Look for terms like sucrose, high fructose corn syrup, cane sugar, and

any word ending in "ose," which typically signifies a sugar. Also, take note of the total grams of sugar in each product.

3. Identify Hidden Sugars: Sugar often hides in unexpected places. Be on the lookout for sugar content in seemingly healthy foods like yogurt, granola bars, salad dressings, and even savory snacks. Note down these sources of hidden sugars in your food diary.

4. Quantify Added Sugar: In your food diary, distinguish between naturally occurring sugars, such as those in fruits and dairy products, and added sugars. Added sugars are those that are not naturally present in the food but are incorporated during processing or preparation.

5. Calculate Daily Intake: At the end of the assessment period, calculate your daily sugar intake by adding up the grams of sugar you consumed each day. Take an average to get a sense of your typical daily sugar consumption.

6. Reflect on Patterns: Review your food diary to identify patterns in your sugar consumption. Do you tend to eat more sugar at certain times of the day or during specific situations, like stress or social gatherings? Recognizing these patterns can help you make targeted changes.

7. Emotional and Social Factors: Consider the emotional and social aspects of your sugar consumption. Are there certain emotions or events that trigger sugar cravings or overindulgence? Understanding the emotional connection to sugar can be crucial for managing it effectively.

8. Set Baseline Goals: With your current sugar intake quantified, set baseline goals for your sugar detox. Decide on a specific reduction target, whether it's cutting your daily sugar intake in half or eliminating all added sugars for a set period.

Assessing your current sugar intake provides you with valuable insights into your dietary habits and helps you establish a clear starting point for your sugar detox journey. Armed with this knowledge, you can set realistic goals, make informed choices, and track your progress effectively as you work towards a healthier, sugar-free lifestyle. Remember that awareness is the first step toward positive change, and your commitment to assessing your sugar intake is a significant stride towards your wellness goals.

Creating a Sugar Detox Shopping List

Creating a Sugar Detox Shopping List is an essential step to ensure you have all the right ingredients to support your journey toward reducing sugar intake. When grocery shopping for your sugar detox, focus on whole, unprocessed foods and prioritize fresh produce, lean proteins, and healthy fats. Here's a complete shopping list to get you started:

Proteins:

- Skinless chicken breast
- Lean turkey
- Salmon or other fatty fish (rich in omega-3 fatty acids)

> Tofu or tempeh (for plant-based options)

> Eggs

> Lean cuts of beef or pork (if desired, in moderation)

Fruits:

✓ Berries (strawberries, blueberries, raspberries)

✓ Apples

✓ Pears

✓ Citrus fruits (oranges, grapefruits)

✓ Avocado (technically a fruit)

✓ Kiwi

✓ Melons (watermelon, cantaloupe)

✓ Tomatoes (technically a fruit)

Vegetables (aim for variety):

• Leafy greens (spinach, kale, arugula)

• Broccoli

• Cauliflower

• Zucchini

• Bell peppers (various colors)

• Cucumbers

- Carrots

- Celery

- Onions

- Garlic

- Sweet potatoes

- Asparagus

- Brussels sprouts

Whole Grains:

- Quinoa

- Brown rice

- Oats (steel-cut or rolled)

- Whole wheat pasta (in moderation)

- Barley

- Bulgur

Nuts and Seeds:

- Almonds

- Walnuts

- Chia seeds

- Flaxseeds

- Sunflower seeds

Dairy or Dairy Alternatives:

- Greek yogurt (unsweetened)
- Unsweetened almond milk, coconut milk, or soy milk (for lactose-free options)
- Cheese (in moderation, if desired)

Fats and Oils:

- Olive oil (extra virgin)
- Coconut oil
- Avocado oil
- Nuts and nut butters (unsweetened)
- Seeds (e.g., flaxseeds, chia seeds)

Herbs, Spices, and Condiments:

- Fresh herbs (e.g., basil, cilantro, parsley)
- Spices (e.g., cinnamon, turmeric, cumin, paprika)
- Vinegar (e.g., balsamic, apple cider vinegar)
- Mustard (unsweetened)
- Salsa (with no added sugars)
- Low-sodium soy sauce or tamari

Beverages:

- Water (hydrate throughout the day)

✓ Herbal teas (no added sugars)

✓ Green tea

✓ Black coffee (if desired, without added sugar)

✓ Sparkling water (unsweetened)

Miscellaneous:

- Legumes (beans, lentils)

- Natural sweeteners (in moderation, if needed): Stevia, monk fruit, erythritol.

- Baking essentials (if you plan to do sugar-free baking): Almond flour, coconut flour, unsweetened cocoa powder

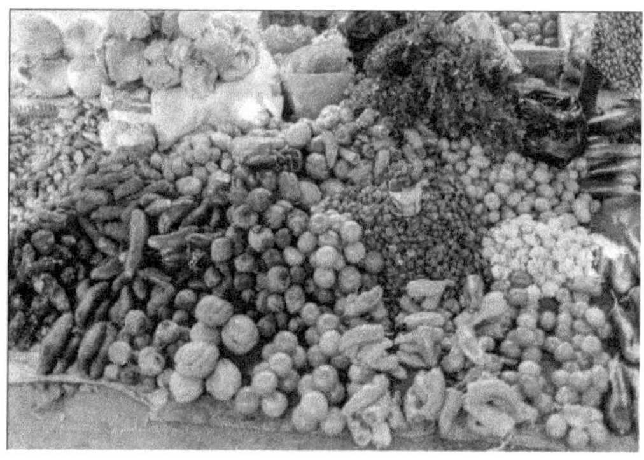

Remember, the key to a successful sugar detox is to avoid or minimize foods with added sugars and refined carbohydrates. Focus on whole, unprocessed foods, and read labels carefully to spot hidden sugars in packaged items. Plan your meals in advance using these ingredients to ensure you have nutritious and satisfying options readily available during your sugar detox journey.

Setting Realistic Goals for Your Journey

In the journey outlined in the Sugar Detox Diet Cookbook, setting realistic goals is a pivotal step toward your success. It's essential to establish clear, attainable objectives that guide you through your sugar detox with purpose and motivation. Here's how to set realistic goals that will keep you on track:

1. Define Your "Why": Start by reflecting on why you're embarking on this sugar detox journey. What motivates you to reduce your sugar intake? Is it weight loss, improved energy, better skin, or overall health? Understanding your "why" will provide a strong foundation for your goals and remind you of

your purpose on days when the journey feels challenging.

2. Make Your Goals Specific: Vague goals can be challenging to measure and achieve. Instead of saying, "I want to reduce my sugar intake," specify exactly what you aim to accomplish. For instance, "I will restrict added sugar to under 25 grams each day" or "I will dispose of sweet snacks from my day to day daily schedule."

3. Be Realistic: While it's admirable to aspire to a sugar-free life, it's essential to set realistic goals that you can maintain. Drastically cutting out all sugar overnight may lead to frustration and potential setbacks. Gradual reductions and sustainable changes are often more effective in the long run.

4. Set Measurable Milestones: Break your sugar detox journey into smaller, measurable milestones. For instance, you might aim to reduce your daily sugar intake by 10 grams per week or eliminate sugary beverages within the first two weeks. Having these smaller goals allows you to track your

progress and celebrate your achievements along the way.

5. Consider a Timeline: Determine a reasonable timeline for your sugar detox. A 30-day detox, as outlined in this cookbook, provides a structured framework and a clear endpoint. However, it's essential to continue setting goals beyond the detox period to maintain your sugar-free lifestyle.

6. Make Goals Actionable: Ensure your goals are actionable and include specific steps you can take to achieve them. Instead of saying, "I want to eat healthier," specify actions like "I will prepare a sugar-free breakfast every morning" or "I will replace sugary snacks with fresh fruit for my afternoon pick-me-up."

7. Stay Flexible: Life is unpredictable, and there may be occasions when adhering to your goals becomes challenging. Be prepared to adapt your goals to suit your circumstances, but always return to your sugar detox plan as soon as possible.

8. Seek Support and Accountability: Share your goals with friends, family, or a support group. Having people who can hold you accountable and provide encouragement can be a powerful motivator.

9. Measure Progress: Regularly assess your progress toward your goals. Keep a journal or use a tracking app to record your daily sugar intake, energy levels, mood, and any physical changes you observe. This tangible evidence of your progress can boost your motivation.

10. Celebrate Achievements: Celebrate your victories, no matter how small. Whether it's reaching a specific milestone or resisting a sugary temptation, acknowledge your efforts and treat yourself to a non-food reward.

Remember that your sugar detox journey is unique to you. Setting realistic goals tailored to your needs and circumstances will make your journey more manageable and sustainable. Embrace the positive changes you're making.

Chapter 2

30-Day Sugar Detox Meal Plan

Week 1: Jumpstart Your Detox with Delicious Smoothie

Day 1: Tropical Paradise Smoothie

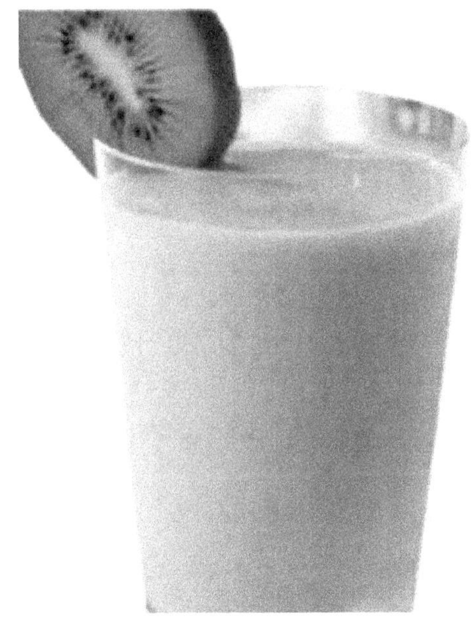

Preparation and cook time: 5-10mins

Ingredients:

1 peeled and chopped ripe mango

1 cup fresh or frozen pineapple chunks

1 banana, ripe

1 cup coconut milk, unsweetened

Ice cubes (optional, depending on desired consistency)

Instructions:

Make the Fruits:

Remove the seed and skin from the mango before peeling and dicing it.

Cut the pineapple into bite-sized chunks.

Combine the following ingredients:

In a blender, combine the mango, pineapple slices, banana, and unsweetened coconut milk.

Blend:

Blend until the mixture is smooth and creamy. If the smoothie is too thick, add a little more water or coconut milk to reach the required consistency.

(Optional): Adjust the sweetness:

Taste the smoothie and, if desired, add a drizzle of honey or a sweetener of your liking. However, because the fruits are sweet by nature, additional sweeteners are frequently unnecessary.

(Optional): Add ice:

Add a handful of ice cubes and blend again until smooth for a cooler, more refreshing smoothie.

Serve:

Pour the smoothie into the glasses and decorate with a slice of pineapple or mango.

Enjoy this tropical Paradise smoothie while it's still fresh and cold.

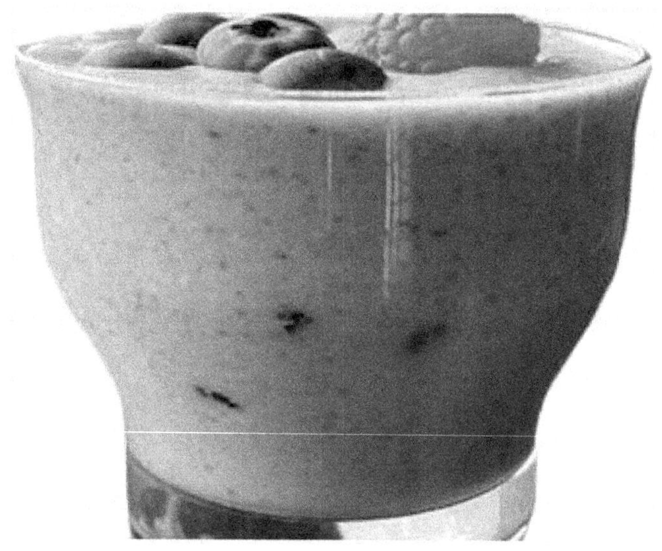

Ingredients:

1 cup fresh or frozen mixed berries (strawberries, blueberries, raspberries, blackberries)

1 banana, ripe

1/2 cup plain Greek yogurt

1/2 cup unsweetened almond milk (or your preferred milk)

1 tbsp honey (optional, for extra sweetness)

1-2 tbsp rolled oats (optional for extra fiber and thickness)

Instructions:

Make the Berries:

If using fresh berries, properly rinse them under cold water and pat them dry. Allow frozen berries to defrost slightly before using.

Combine the following ingredients:

Blend the mixed berries, ripe banana, Greek yogurt, unsweetened almond milk, honey (if used), and rolled oats together in a blender.

Blend:

Blend until the mixture is smooth and creamy. If the smoothie is too thick, you may thin it up with a little more almond milk or water.

(Optional): Adjust the sweetness:

If you prefer a sweeter taste, add extra honey to the smoothie. Remember that the sweetness of the fruits may enough.

(Optional): Add ice:

Add a handful of ice cubes and blend again until smooth for a cooler, more refreshing smoothie.

Serve:

Fill a glass halfway with the Berry Blast Breakfast Smoothie.

(Optional garnish):

For an eye-catching display, garnish with a few whole berries or a mint leaf.

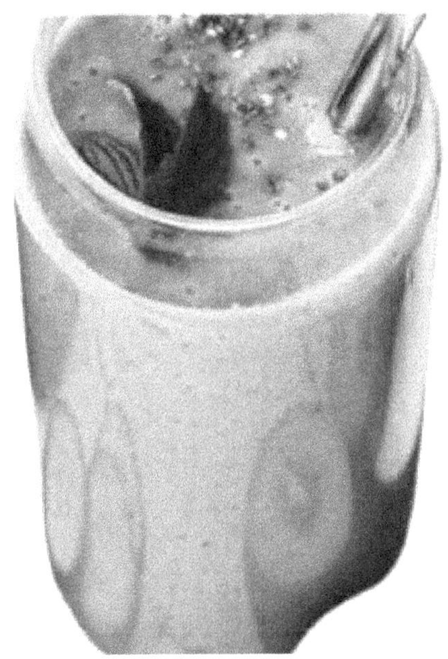

Ingredients

1 cup spinach (either fresh or frozen)

1/2 cup fresh or frozen kale

1/2 cucumber, diced

a half avocado

1 green apple, peeled and cut

1 lemon (juiced)

1 inch piece peeled fresh ginger

1-2 cups water or unsweetened almond milk

Ice cubes are optional.

Instructions:

Gather the Ingredients:

Begin by thoroughly cleaning all of the fruits and vegetables. Cut the cucumber, green apple, and avocado into bite-sized pieces.

Mix the Greens:

Blend spinach, kale, cucumber, and green apple in a blender. Blend until completely smooth.

Mix in the avocado and lemon:

To the combined greens, add the avocado, lemon juice, and peeled ginger. Blend until smooth and creamy again.

Consistency should be adjusted:

To reach the ideal smoothie consistency, gradually add almond milk or water. Blend until all of the ingredients are well incorporated.

Adjust to taste:

Adjust the sweetness or sharpness of the smoothie by adding extra lemon juice or a tiny bit of honey/agave syrup as needed.

Serve:

Pour the smoothie into a glass and top with ice cubes if preferred for a refreshing coolness.

(Optional garnish):

For a decorative touch, garnish with a slice of lemon or a few cucumber slices.

As a healthy and rejuvenating treat, try this green energy sugar detox smoothie!

Day 4: Creamy Chocolate Avocado Smoothie

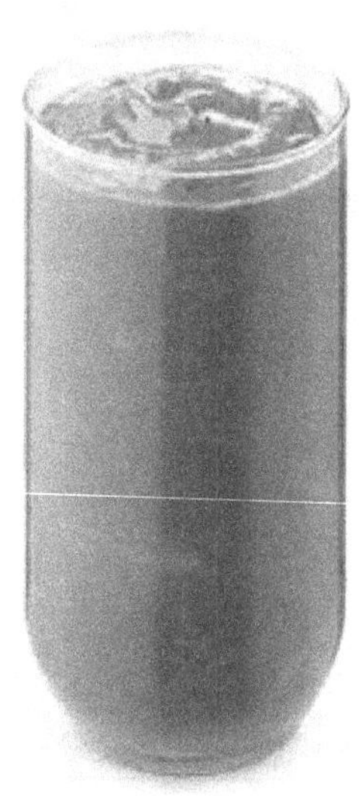

Ingredients:

1 ripe avocado

1 ripe banana

2 tablespoons unsweetened cocoa powder

1/2 teaspoon pure vanilla extract

1-2 tablespoons of a natural sweetener (like honey, maple syrup, or agave nectar), to taste

1 cup unsweetened almond milk (or any preferred milk)

1/2 cup Greek yogurt (optional for added creaminess)

1-2 cups ice cubes

A pinch of salt

Instructions:

Prepare the Ingredients:

Start by peeling and removing the pit from the avocado and banana. Make sure they are ripe for a creamy texture.

Blend the Ingredients:

In a blender, combine the avocado, banana, unsweetened cocoa powder, vanilla extract, your chosen sweetener (start with a smaller amount and adjust to your taste), almond milk, Greek yogurt (if using), and a pinch of salt.

Blend Until Smooth:

Blend the ingredients until you achieve a smooth and creamy consistency. If the mixture is too thick, you can add more almond milk as needed.

Taste and Adjust:

Taste the smoothie and adjust the sweetness, as well as the cocoa flavor to your liking. Add more sweetener or cocoa powder if necessary.

Add Ice and Blend:

Add 1-2 cups of ice cubes to the blender and blend again until the smoothie is well-chilled and has a thick, milkshake-like consistency.

Serve:

Pour the creamy chocolate avocado sugar detox smoothie into a glass.

Optional Garnishes:

If desired, you can top the smoothie with grated dark chocolate, a dollop of Greek yogurt, or a sprinkle of unsweetened cocoa powder

Day 5: Refreshing Cucumber Mint Smoothie

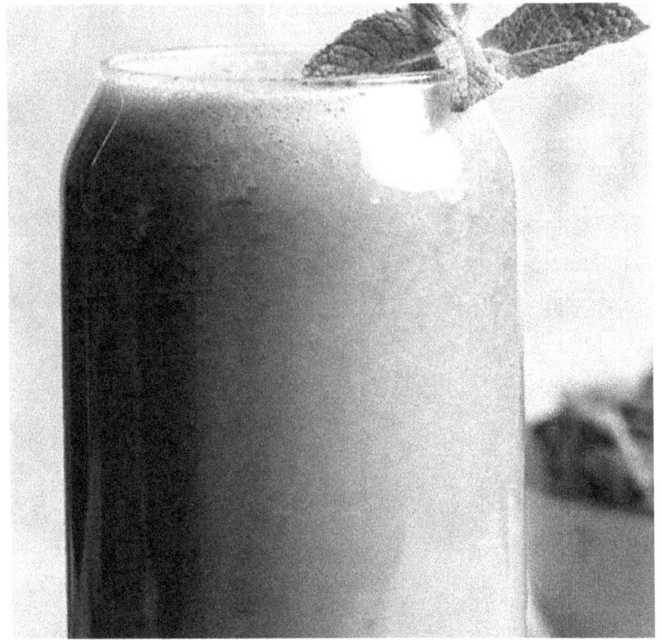

Ingredients:

1 big peeled and sliced cucumber

1 cup spinach leaves, fresh

1/2 cup mint leaves, fresh

1 lemon (juiced)

1/2 cup plain Greek yogurt (or dairy-free equivalent)

1/2 cup unsweetened almond milk (or unsweetened milk of choice)

Optional:

1/2 teaspoon fresh grated ginger

Optional ice cubes (for added cold)

Sugar-free sweetener (to taste)

Instructions:

1. Gather Your Ingredients:

Wash and peel the cucumber before cutting it into slices.

Thoroughly wash the spinach and mint leaves.

The lemon should be juiced.

Grate your fresh ginger, if you would like to use it.

2. Combine the ingredients:

Blend the cucumber, fresh spinach leaves, mint leaves, lemon juice, Greek yogurt, almond milk, and ginger (if using) in a blender.

3. Blend till smooth:

Begin by blending the ingredients on low speed and gradually increasing to high speed.

Blend until smooth and all of the components are fully incorporated. If you want a cooler smoothie, add some ice cubes.

4. Taste and Modify:

Adjust the sweetness or tanginess of the smoothie by adding extra lemon juice or sugar as desired.

5. Serve and Have Fun:

Fill a glass halfway with the smoothie.

If desired, garnish with a mint leaf or a cucumber slice.

Have fun with your delicious Cucumber Mint Smoothie!

This smoothie is ideal for a sugar detox since it includes no additional sweets and is packed with hydrating cucumber, nutrient-rich spinach, and the refreshing flavor of mint. It's a nutritious and tasty way to start the day or as a snack.

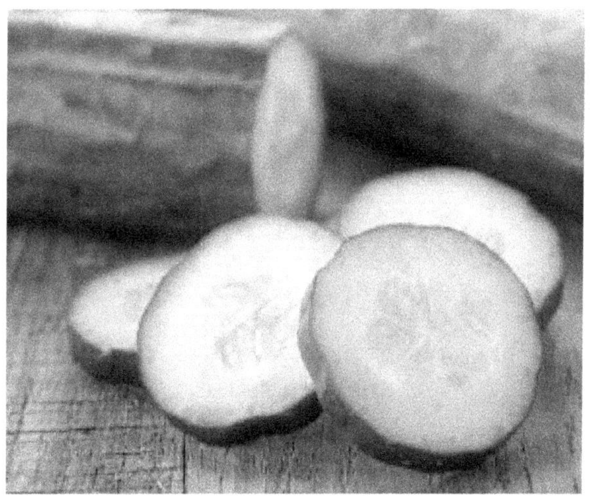

Ingredients:

2 big peeled and segmented oranges

1/2 cup plain Greek yogurt (or a dairy-free substitute)

1/2 cup unsweetened almond milk (or unsweetened milk of choice)

1 teaspoon vanilla essence, pure

1 tsp grated orange zest (optional, for added taste)

Optional ice cubes (for added cold)

Instructions:

1. Gather Your Ingredients:

Remove the peel off the oranges and cut them into segments. Remove any seeds that may be present.

2. Combine the ingredients:

Blend the orange segments, unsweetened Greek yogurt, unsweetened almond milk, vanilla extract, and grated orange zest (if used) in a blender until smooth.

If you want a colder and frostier smoothie, add ice cubes.

3. Puree till smooth:

Begin blending on low to break down the ingredients, then gradually raise to high speed.

Blend until smooth and all of the components are fully incorporated.

4. Taste and Modify:

Adjust the flavor and consistency of the smoothie as needed. If you want it sweeter, add a pinch of stevia or a sugar-free sweetener.

5. Serve and Have Fun:

Fill a glass halfway with Orange Dreamsicle Smoothie.

For an added flavor boost, garnish with a tiny orange slice or a sprinkle of grated orange zest.

Have fun with your sugar-free Orange Dreamsicle Smoothie!

This smoothie has a citrus flavor explosion without any additional sweeteners. Oranges have a natural sweetness to them, and the Greek yogurt provides creaminess and protein to keep you satiated. It's an excellent solution for individuals who want to limit their sugar intake while still enjoying a tasty and refreshing beverage.

Day 7: Detoxifying Blueberry Lemonade Smoothie

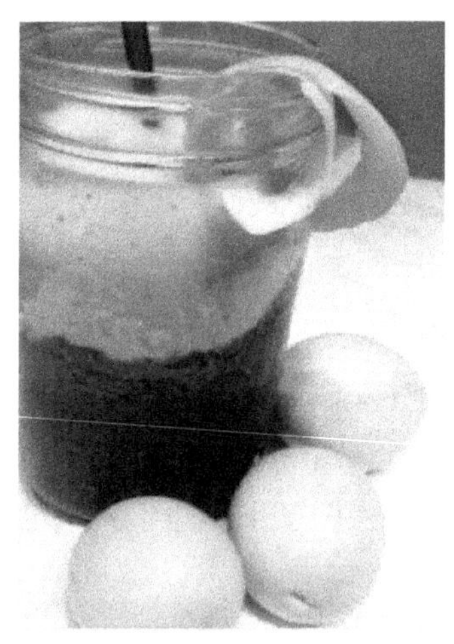

Ingredients:

1 cup blueberries, fresh or frozen

1 lemon juice

1/2 cup plain Greek yogurt (or dairy-free equivalent)

1/2 cup unsweetened almond milk (or unsweetened milk of choice)

1 teaspoon chia seeds

Optional: 1/2 teaspoon fresh grated ginger

Optional ice cubes (for added cold)

Stevia or another sugar-free sweetener (to taste)

Instructions:

1. Gather Your Ingredients:

If using fresh blueberries, properly wash them. Allow frozen blueberries to defrost slightly before using.

The lemon should be juiced.

If you are using fresh ginger, grate it.

2. Blend the ingredients:

Blend the blueberries, lemon juice, plain Greek yogurt, unsweetened almond milk, chia seeds, and grated ginger (if using) in a blender until smooth.

You may add a little bit of Stevia or another sugar-free sweetener of your choice if you like a sweeter taste without additional sugars. Add in small quantity and gradually increase to taste.

3. Puree till smooth:

Begin by blending the ingredients on low speed and gradually increasing to high speed.

Blend until smooth and all of the components are fully incorporated. If you want a cooler smoothie, add some ice cubes.

4. Taste and Modify:

Adjust the sweetness or sharpness of the smoothie by adding extra lemon juice or sugar as desired.

5. Serve and Have Fun:

Fill a glass halfway with the Detoxifying Blueberry Lemonade Smoothie.

If preferred, top with a slice of lemon or a few fresh blueberries.

As part of your sugar detox, try this refreshing and purifying smoothie!

This smooth includes no additional sweets and is wonderfully refreshing due to the natural sweetness of blueberries and the acidity of lemon. The fiber and good fats provided by the chia seeds make it a delicious and nutritious alternative for a detox program.

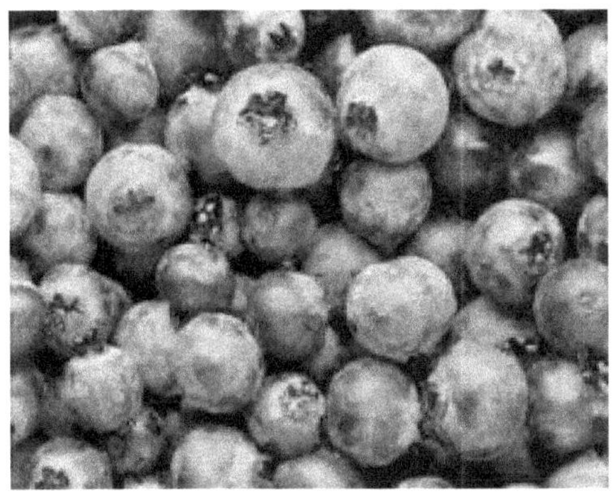

BLUEBERRY

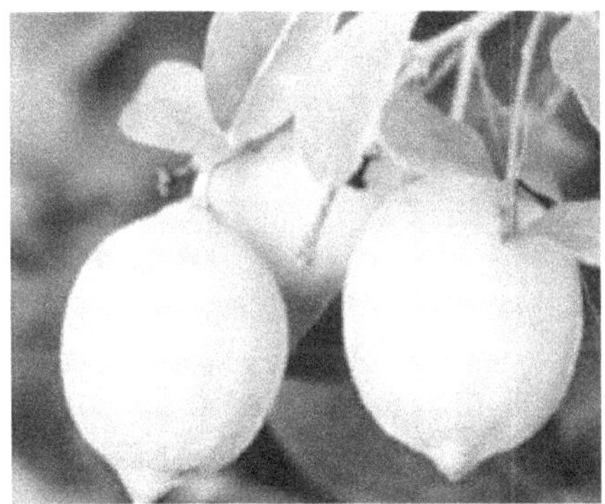

Day 8: Veggie-Packed Breakfast Scramble

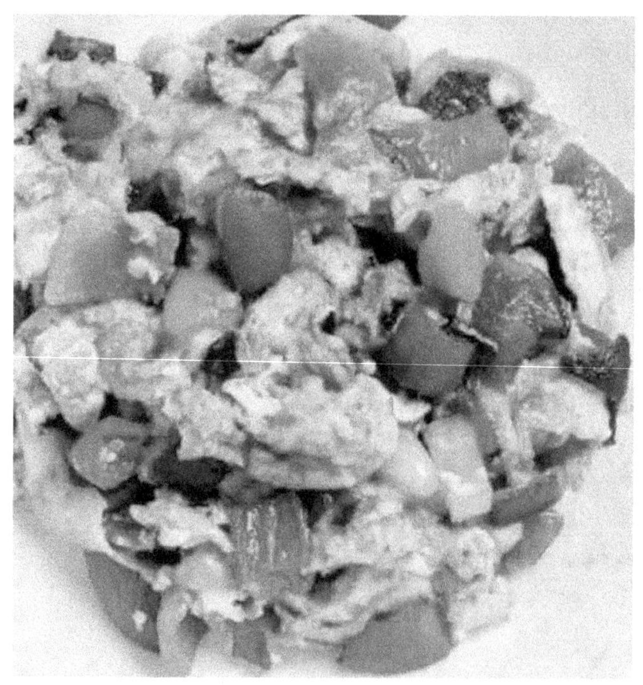

Ingredients:

Two huge eggs

1/4 cup chopped red, yellow, or green bell peppers

A quarter cup chopped tomatoes

1/4 cup red onion, chopped

1/4 cup spinach or kale, chopped

1/4 cup mushrooms, sliced

1/4 cup zucchini, diced

Optional: 1/4 cup diced avocado

1 tablespoon olive oil

Season with salt and pepper to taste.

Garnish with fresh herbs like as parsley or cilantro, if desired.

Instructions:

1. Gather Your Ingredients:

All veggies should be washed and chopped as needed.

Set aside any avocado that has been diced.

2. Heat the Pan:

Heat a non-stick pan over medium heat and add the olive oil.

3. Sauté the Vegetables:

Add the diced red onions, bell peppers, and mushrooms to the skillet. Sauté for 2-3 minutes until they start to soften.

4. Add Zucchini and Tomatoes:

To the skillet, add the diced zucchini and tomatoes.

Cook for another 2-3 minutes, or until the zucchini is cooked and the tomatoes have softened somewhat.

5. Include spinach or kale:

Cook for a further 1-2 minutes or until the spinach or kale has wilted.

6. Make the scrambled eggs:

Transfer the sautéed vegetables to one side of the skillet.

Scramble the eggs on the empty side of the skillet using a spatula.

7. Mix and season:

When the eggs are almost done, combine them with the sautéed veggies.

Season the scramble to taste with salt and pepper.

8. Optional: Add avocado:

If using avocado, carefully mix the cubed avocado into the scramble.

9. Garnish and serve:

Place the Veggie-Packed Breakfast Scramble on a serving platter.

You can also garnish with fresh herbs such as parsley or cilantro.

This Veggie-Packed Breakfast Scramble is a delightful and nutritious option because It's high in fiber and critical nutrients from a variety of veggies, and it gives a satisfying start to the day without the need of added sweets. It's also a versatile dish, so feel free to experiment with your favorite vegetables.

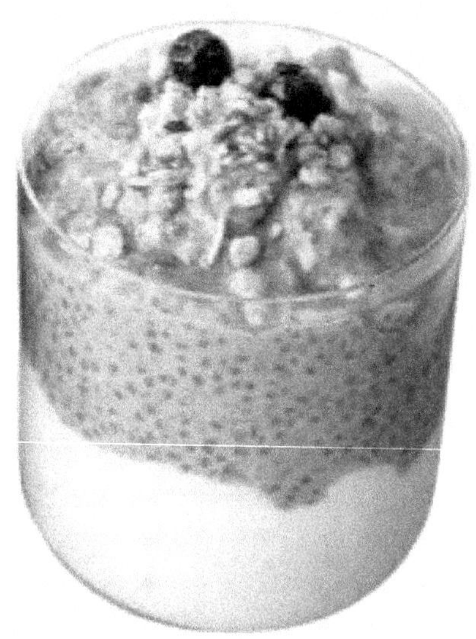

Ingredients

To prepare the Chia Seed Pudding:

Three tbsp chia seeds

1 cup unsweetened almond milk (or your favorite unsweetened milk)

1/2 tsp pure vanilla extract

1-2 teaspoons sugar-free sweetener such as stevia or erythritol (to taste)

Optional: a pinch of cinnamon

To make the Berry Topping:

1/2 cup mixed berries (strawberries, blueberries, raspberries, etc.)

a dab of freshly squeezed lemon juice

Garnish with fresh mint leaves (optional).

Instructions:

1. Gather Your Ingredients:

If necessary, wash and cut the mixed berries.

Squeeze fresh lemon juice over the berries and mix gently.

2. Whip up the Chia Seed Pudding:

Combine the chia seeds, unsweetened almond milk, pure vanilla extract, sugar-free sweetener, and cinnamon (if using) in a mixing dish.

To blend, thoroughly stir the mixture.

3. Combine and Set:

Make sure there are no clumps in the chia seed pudding mixture.

Place the bowl of chia seed in the fridge for at least 4 hours or overnight. The chia seeds will absorb the liquid and form a pudding-like consistency during this time.

4. Put everything together and serve:

Spoon the chia pudding into serving plates or jars after it has set.

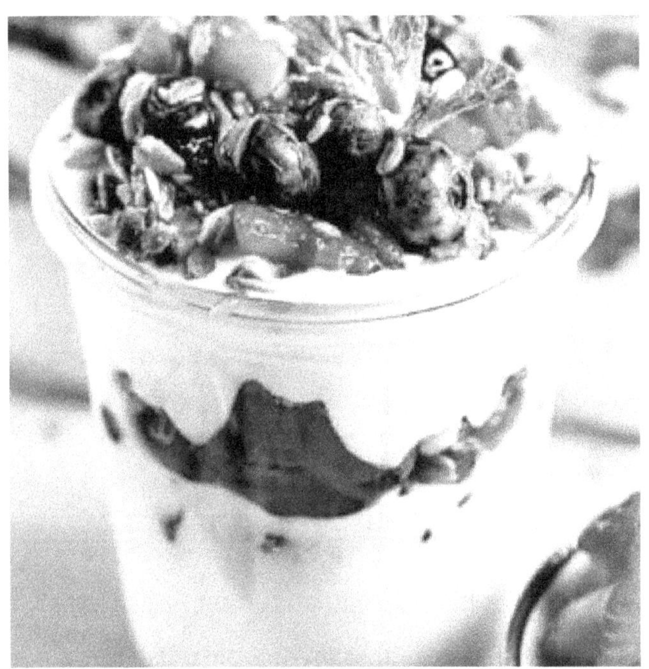

Ingredients:

1 cup plain (unsweetened) Greek yogurt

1/2 cup berries (strawberries, blueberries, raspberries, etc.)

1/4 cup unsweetened granola or chopped nuts (almonds or walnuts, for example)

1 teaspoon vanilla essence, pure

Optional: a drizzle of sugar-free honey or a sugar-free sweetener

Garnish with fresh mint leaves (optional).

Instructions:

1. Gather Your Ingredients:

If necessary, wash and cut the mixed berries.

If you're using nuts, break them up into smaller bits.

2. Optionally sweeten the Greek yogurt:

Combine the plain Greek yogurt and a teaspoon of pure vanilla essence in a mixing dish. If you want to add more sweetness, sprinkle with sugar-free honey or a sugar-free sweetener. Adapt to your personal tastes.

3. Make the Parfait:

Begin by putting the sweetened Greek yogurt at the bottom of a glass or dish.

4. Include Berries:

On top of the yogurt, put a layer of mixed berries.

5. Sprinkle with granola or nuts:

Sprinkle the berries with unsweetened granola or chopped almonds. This provides texture as well as a pleasing crunch.

6. Repetition of Layers:

If your serving dish has additional room, you can repeat the layers, beginning with yogurt and finishing with berries and granola or nuts.

7. Add a garnish:

Garnish your Greek Yogurt Parfait with fresh mint leaves if desired for a splash of color and taste.

This Greek Yogurt Parfait is an excellent choice for a sugar detox diet. It has a lot of protein, probiotics (from the yogurt), fiber (from the berries), and healthy fats (from the almonds). The berries' inherent sweetness lends a hint of sweetness without the need of additional sweeteners. Enjoy it as a nutritious and tasty breakfast or snack.

Day 11: Sweet Potato Hash

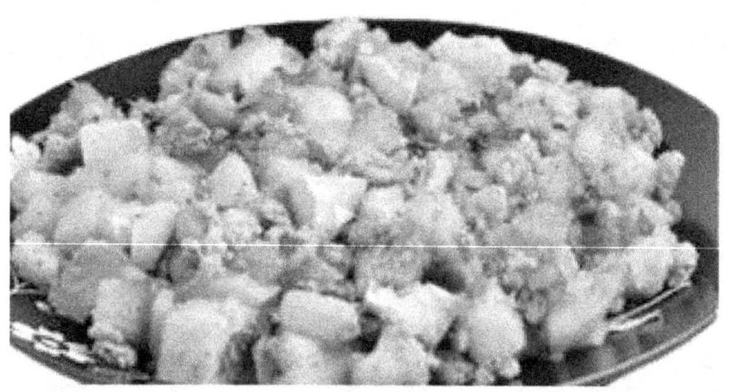

Ingredients:

2 medium peeled and sliced sweet potatoes into tiny pieces

1 finely chopped tiny red onion

1 chopped red bell pepper

1 diced green bell pepper

2 minced garlic cloves

2 tbsp olive oil (or coconut oil)

1 paprika teaspoon

1/2 teaspoon cumin powder

Season with salt and black pepper to taste.

Garnish with fresh parsley or cilantro (optional).

Instructions:

1. Gather Your Ingredients:

Sweet potatoes should be peeled and diced into tiny, even pieces.

Chop the red onion finely.

Cut the red and green bell peppers into dice.

Garlic should be minced.

2. Peel and parboil the sweet potatoes:

Parboil the sweet potato cubes in a saucepan of boiling water for about 5-7 minutes, or until they're somewhat soft but not totally cooked. Set aside after draining.

3. Cook the Vegetables:

Heat the olive oil or coconut oil in a large pan over medium-high heat.

Mix in the red onion and garlic. Sauté for a few minutes, or until they begin to smell pleasant.

4. Stir in the sweet potatoes and bell peppers:

To the pan, add the parboiled sweet potatoes and red and green bell peppers.

Cook, tossing periodically, for approximately 10-15 minutes, or until the sweet potatoes are golden brown and crispy on the exterior and the peppers are soft.

Seasonings and spices:

Sprinkle the sweet potato mixture with paprika, cumin, salt, and black pepper.

Stir well to coat the veggies evenly with the seasonings.

Cooking Time: 6 minutes

Cook for 5-10 minutes more, stirring periodically, until the sweet potatoes are thoroughly cooked and crispy.

7. Decorate and serve:

Place the Sweet Potato Hash in a serving bowl.

If preferred, garnish with fresh parsley or cilantro.

Sweet potatoes are naturally sweet and include a good amount of carbs and fiber. Without the use of added sweets, the bright bell peppers and aromatic spices provide a wonderful touch to this recipe. Serve it as a filling breakfast or as a nutritious side dish for lunch or supper.

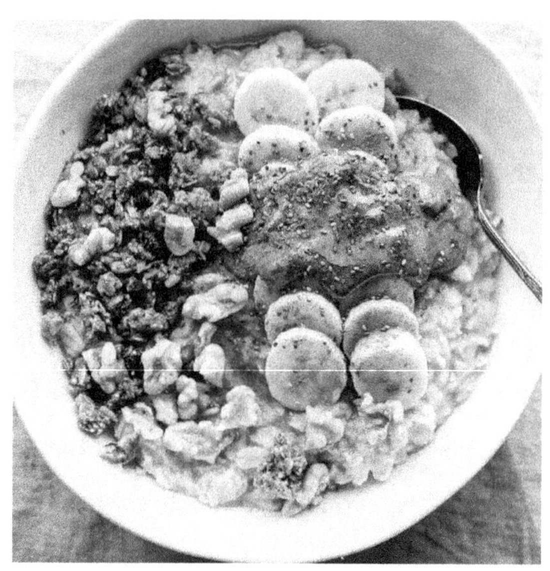

Ingredients:

1/2 cup rolled oats (gluten-free if necessary)

1 cup unsweetened almond milk (or your favorite unsweetened milk)

1 mashed ripe banana

1-2 tbsp unsweetened almond butter

1/2 tsp pure vanilla extract

a pinch of cinnamon powder

Optional garnish: sliced almonds

Instructions:

1. Prepare the Oatmeal:

Combine the rolled oats and unsweetened almond milk in a saucepan.

Over medium heat, bring the mixture to a moderate simmer.

2. Mash the banana:

Add the mashed ripe banana after the oats begin to boil and thicken (approximately 2-3 minutes).

3. Continue to Cook:

Stir thoroughly and heat, stirring occasionally, until the oatmeal is the appropriate consistency. This typically takes 5-7 minutes.

4. Taste and sweetness

To the oatmeal, mix in almond butter, pure vanilla essence, and a sprinkle of ground cinnamon.

Stir together until everything is properly combined.

5. Garnish and serve:

Place the Almond Butter Banana Oatmeal in a mixing dish.

Garnish with chopped almonds for added texture and a nutty taste if preferred.

This Almond Butter Banana Oatmeal is a tasty, sugar-free breakfast choice. The natural sweetness of ripe bananas offers all the sweetness you want without the use of extra sweeteners. The almond butter offers a creamy texture and healthful fats, while the oats provide fiber to keep you full. As part of your sugar detox strategy, enjoy this nourishing and cozy breakfast.

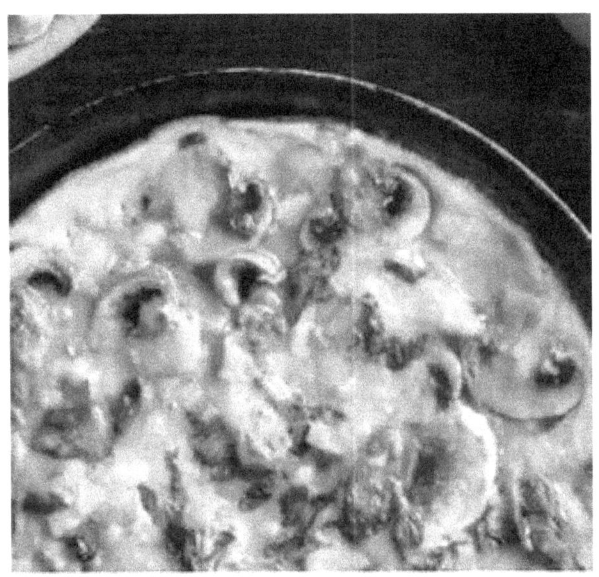

Ingredients:

Two huge eggs

1 cup spinach leaves, fresh

1/2 cup mushrooms, sliced

1/4 cup chopped red bell pepper 1/4 cup diced onion

1 minced garlic clove

1 tablespoon extra virgin olive oil

Season with salt and black pepper to taste.

Use fresh herbs such as parsley or chives to garnish (optional).

Instructions:

1. Gather Your Ingredients:

Drain any extra water from the fresh spinach leaves.

The mushrooms should be sliced, the onion and red bell pepper diced, and the garlic minced.

2. Cook the Vegetables:

Heat the olive oil in a nonstick skillet over medium-high heat.

Sauté the chopped onion and minced garlic for a couple of minutes, or until fragrant.

3. Mix in the mushrooms and red bell pepper:

In the skillet, add the sliced mushrooms and chopped red bell pepper.

Sauté the veggies for 5-7 minutes, or until the liquid from the mushrooms has evaporated.

4. Add the spinach:

Cook for a further 2-3 minutes, or until the new spinach leaves are wilted.

5. The season:

Season the vegetable combination to taste with salt and black pepper. Set aside the cooked veggies.

6. Make the Omelette:

In a mixing dish, combine the two big eggs.

7. Prepare the Omelette:

If necessary, add a little extra olive oil to the same skillet.

Pour the beaten eggs into the skillet and leave them to simmer for a minute or two, stirring occasionally.

8. Include Vegetables:

Spread the cooked vegetable mixture equally over one-half of the omelette after the eggs are halfway set.

9. Fold and plate:

Fold the second half of the omelette gently over the veggies to form a half-moon shape.

Cook for 1 minute, or until the eggs are fully set.

10. Decorate and serve:

- Serve the Spinach and Mushroom Omelette with fresh herbs such as parsley or chives, if preferred.

This Spinach and Mushroom Omelette is a filling and tasty meal that contains no added sweeteners. It's high in protein, vitamins, and minerals thanks to the veggies and eggs, making it a good choice for a sugar detox diet. Start your day off right with this nutritious and tasty omelette.

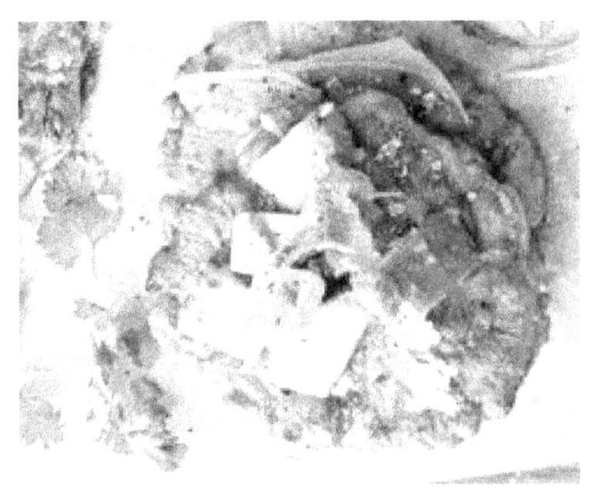

Ingredients:

For the Zucchini Fritters, combine the following ingredients:

2 medium grated zucchinis

1 teaspoon of salt

1/4 cup almond flour (or your favorite sugar-free flour)

1/4 cup grated Parmesan cheese (optional; if preferred, use a dairy-free substitute)

1/4 cup fresh herbs, chopped (parsley, chives, or cilantro)

2 minced garlic cloves

1 big egg 1 tablespoon olive oil for frying

To make the Avocado Salsa:

1 ripe avocado, diced 1 small tomato, diced 1/4 cup red onion, finely chopped 1/4 cup fresh cilantro, chopped

Season with salt and pepper to taste.

Instructions:

1. Gather Your Ingredients:

Place the zucchinis in a colander and grate them. Sprinkle with salt and let aside for 10 minutes. This can help in the removing excess moisture.

2 Prepare the Avocado Salsa:

Prepare the avocado salsa while the zucchinis drain. Combine the chopped avocado, tomato, red onion, cilantro, lime juice, salt, and pepper in a mixing bowl. Toss gently to mix. Set aside the salsa.

3. Drain and squeeze the zucchini:

Squeeze the shredded zucchinis to eliminate extra liquid after 10 minutes. You may do this using a clean kitchen towel or paper towels.

4. Make the fritter batter:

Combine the drained zucchinis, almond flour, grated Parmesan cheese (if using), and chopped herbs, minced garlic, and the egg in a large mixing dish. Mix until the mixture is cohesive.

5. Prepare the Fritters:

Heat a tiny quantity of olive oil in a pan over medium heat.

Scoop out parts of the zucchini mixture with a spoon and flatten them into fritters in the pan.

Cook for 3-4 minutes on each side, or until golden brown and crisp. You might have to cook them in batches.

6. Serve:

Serve the Zucchini Fritters with the prepared Avocado Salsa.

These Zucchini Fritters with Avocado Salsa are a tasty and filling sugar-free supper. Zucchinis are naturally low in sugar and high in fiber, while the avocado salsa provides healthy fats and a flavorful burst. It's a nutrient-dense, sugar-free solution for sugar detoxing women.

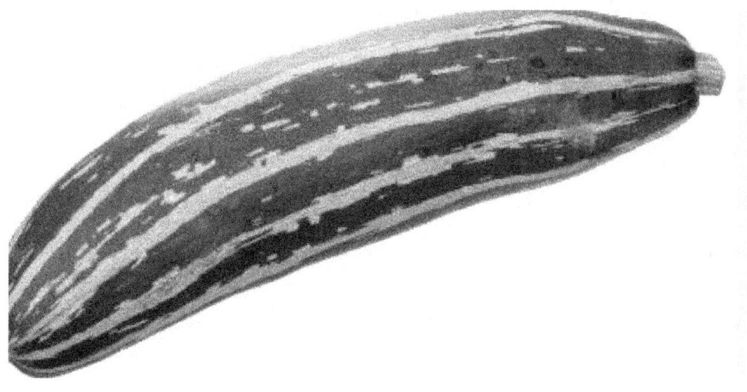

ZUCCHINI

Day 15: Quinoa and Chickpea Salad

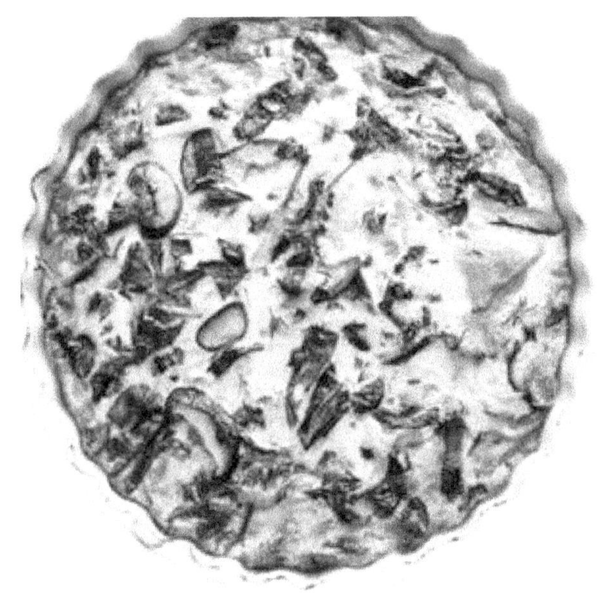

Ingredients:

Salad Ingredients:

1 cup washed and cooked quinoa, according to package directions

1 can (15 oz) drained and rinsed chickpeas (or 1.5 cups cooked chickpeas)

1 cup cucumber, diced

1 cup red bell pepper, chopped

1/2 cup red onion, chopped

1/4 cup fresh parsley, chopped

Optional: 1/4 cup chopped fresh mint

1/4 cup crumbled feta cheese (optional; substitute a dairy-free version if preferred)

To make the dressing:

3 tbsp extra virgin olive oil

2 tbsp. fresh lemon juice

1 minced garlic clove

1/2 teaspoon cumin powder

Season with salt and black pepper to taste.

Instructions:

1. Gather Your Ingredients:

Cook the quinoa according per the package directions after rinsing it under cool water. Allow to cool after cooking.

2. Prepare the Dressing:

Whisk together the extra-virgin olive oil, fresh lemon juice, minced garlic, ground cumin, salt, and black pepper in a small bowl. Set aside the dressing.

3. Mix together the salad ingredients:

Combine the cooked quinoa, chickpeas, diced cucumber, diced red bell pepper, diced red onion, chopped fresh parsley, and chopped fresh mint (if using) in a large mixing dish.

4. Drizzle with dressing:

Pour the dressing over the salad items and toss to combine.

5. Chill and Toss:

Toss the salad gently to mix all of the ingredients and coat them with the dressing.

Refrigerate the salad for 30 minutes to enable the flavors to combine.

6. Optional garnish:

Before serving, put crumbled feta cheese on top of the salad if preferred.

This Quinoa and Chickpea Salad is a nutritious, well-balanced, and sugar-free dinner. Quinoa and chickpeas are high in protein and fiber, while the colorful veggies are high in vitamins and minerals. The fresh herbs and spicy dressing complement the tastes without adding any sweetness. As part of your sugar detox strategy, use this salad as a filling lunch or supper choice.

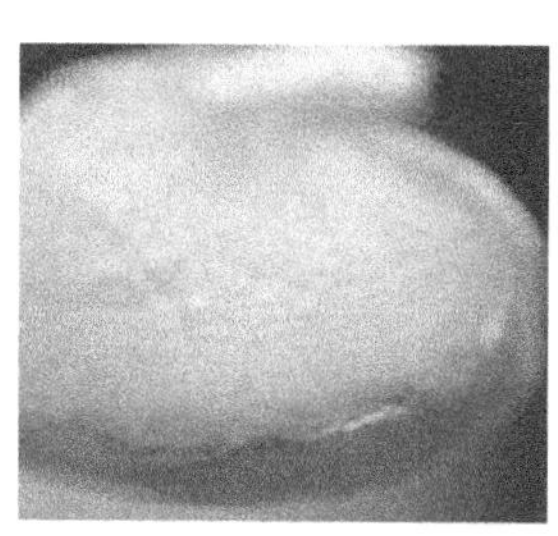

QUINOA SEED

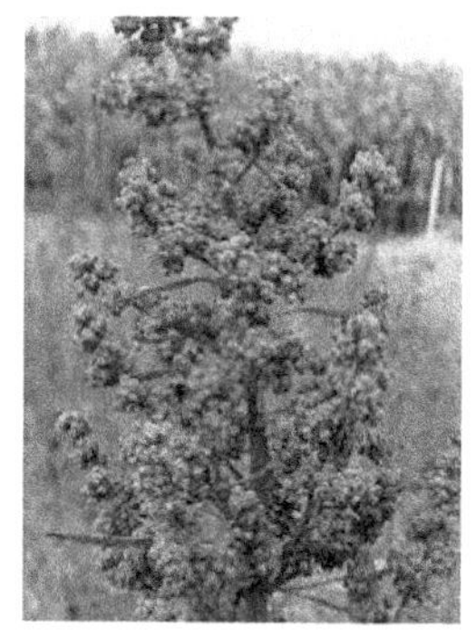

QUINOA FLOWERS

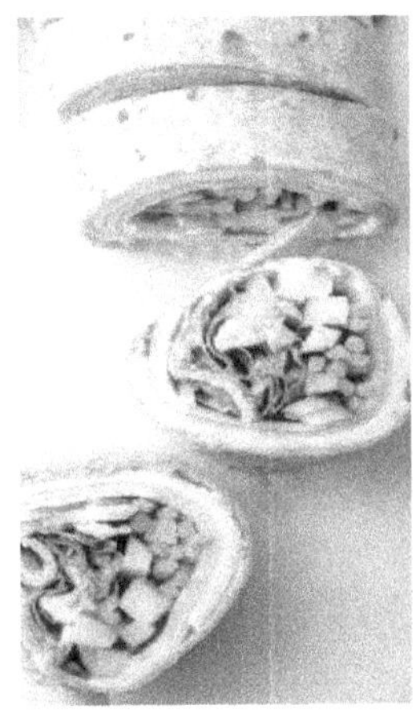

Ingredients:

For the Wrap:

1 whole-grain or whole-wheat tortilla (no added sugars preferred)

4-6 lean turkey breast slices

1/4 cup hummus (preferably sugar-free)

1/2 cup fresh veggies (sliced cucumber, red bell pepper, shredded carrots, spinach)

1/4 sliced avocado

1 chopped small tomato

Sprouts (such as alfalfa sprouts) for crunch and taste

Add salt and black pepper to taste.

To make the dressing (optional):

1 tbsp olive oil (extra virgin)

1 tbsp. balsamic vinegar

1/2 teaspoon sugar-free Dijon mustard

1 teaspoon dried oregano

Add salt and black pepper to taste.

Instructions:

1. Gather Your Ingredients:

All of your fresh veggies should be washed, sliced, and prepared.

2. (Optional) Make the Dressing:

Whisk together the extra-virgin olive oil, balsamic vinegar, Dijon mustard, dried oregano, salt, and black pepper in a small bowl. If you want to use the dressing, set it aside.

3. Put the Wrap Together:

Place a whole-grain or whole-wheat tortilla on a clean surface.

4. Distribute Hummus:

Spread hummus evenly on the tortilla.

5. Add the turkey and vegetables:

Place the hummus on top of the lean turkey breast pieces.

Combine the fresh veggies, avocado slices, tomato slices, and sprouts in a mixing bowl.

6. Season:

Season the veggies to taste with salt and black pepper.

7. Optional Drizzle with Dressing:

Drizzle the dressing over the vegetables if using.

8. Concluding Remarks:

Fold in the edges of the tortilla carefully, then roll it up firmly to make the wrap.

9. Serve and Have Fun:

To make it simpler to handle, cut the Turkey and Veggie Wrap in half.

Serve and enjoy a delectable and sugar-free dinner.

This Turkey and Veggie Wrap is a nutrient-dense, well-balanced, and sugar-free choice. It contains lean turkey protein, healthy fats from avocado, and a range of vitamins and minerals from fresh veggies. As part of your sugar detox strategy, serve it as a filling and nutritious lunch or dinner.

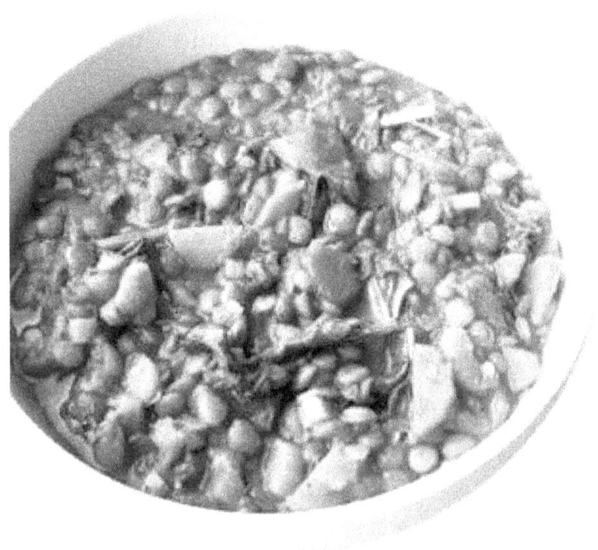

Ingredients:

One cup washed and drained brown lentils or dry green

1 chopped onion

2 minced garlic cloves

2 sliced carrots

2 diced celery stalks

1 cup chopped tomatoes (fresh or canned)

1 teaspoon ground cumin six cups low-sodium vegetable broth

1/2 teaspoon coriander powder

1 teaspoon turmeric powder

1/2 teaspoon paprika powder

Add salt and black pepper to taste.

4 cups chopped fresh spinach

1 lemon juice

Optional olive oil for sautéing

Garnish with fresh parsley or cilantro (optional).

Instructions:

1. Sauté the Aromatics (if using):

Warm a little olive oil in a large soup pot over medium heat. If you prefer an oil-free soup, sauté in a little water or veggie broth instead.

Combine the onion, garlic, carrots, and celery. Cook for 5 minutes, or until the veggies soften and the onions turn translucent.

2. Seasonings:

Combine the ground cumin, ground coriander, ground turmeric, and ground paprika in a mixing bowl. Cook for 1-2 minutes, or until the spices are aromatic.

3. Combine the lentils and the broth:

Pour in the rinsed lentils and diced tomatoes. Combine the sautéed veggies and seasonings in a mixing bowl.

Pour in the vegetable broth with reduced sodium content.

4. Simmering:

Bring the soup to a boil, then lower to a low heat and cook for 25-30 minutes, or until the lentils are cooked.

5. The season:

Add salt and black pepper in the soup to taste.

6. Add the spinach:

Stir in the chopped fresh spinach and allow it to wilt in the heated soup for a minute or two.

7. Finish with a squeeze of lemon juice:

Squeeze one lemon's juice into the soup and whisk to combine.

8. Decorate and serve:

Pour the Lentil Soup with Spinach into serving dishes.

Garnish with fresh parsley or cilantro if preferred.

This Lentil Soup with Spinach is a filling and sugar-free option. Lentils are high in protein and fiber, while spinach provides vitamins and minerals. The fragrant spices offer taste without the need of additional sweeteners. As part of your sugar detox strategy, enjoy this soup as a filling and pleasant dinner.

Day 18: Salmon and Avocado Salad

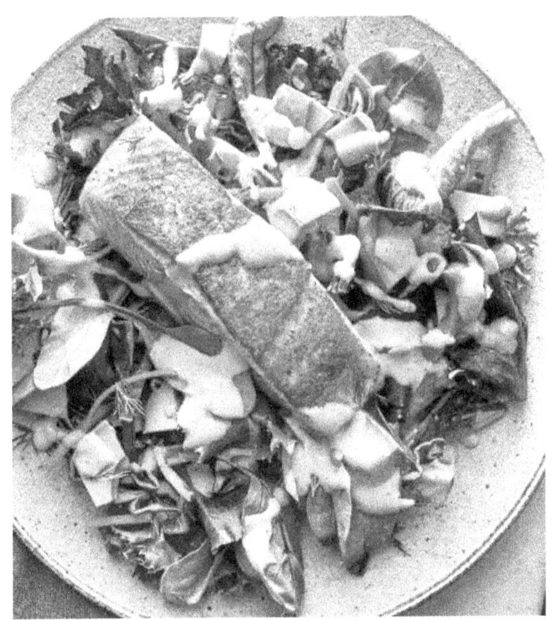

Ingredients:

Salad Ingredients:

2 cooked and flaked salmon fillets (baked, grilled, or poached)

4 cups salad greens (spinach, arugula, or spring mix)

1/4 cup toasted nut pieces 1 ripe avocado, cut 1/2 cucumber, thinly sliced 1/4 red onion, thinly sliced Cherry tomatoes, halved

Optional garnish: fresh dill

To make the dressing:

2 tbsp extra virgin olive oil

1 tablespoon freshly squeezed lemon juice

1 minced garlic clove

Add salt and black pepper to taste.

Instructions:

1. Gather Your Ingredients:

Cook the salmon fillets according to your preference (roasted, grilled, or poached) until flaky. Leave to cool before flaking into bite-sized pieces.

Cut the ripe avocado, cucumber, and red onion into slices.

Cut the cherry tomatoes in half.

Toast the almond pieces until they are golden brown.

2. Prepare the Dressing:

Whisk together the extra-virgin olive oil, fresh lemon juice, minced garlic, salt, and black pepper in a small bowl. Set aside the dressing.

3. Prepare the Salad:

Arrange the mixed salad greens as the basis in a large salad bowl.

4. Include salmon and vegetables:

Top the greens with the flakes salmon.

Combine the avocado, cucumber, red onion, and cherry tomatoes in a mixing bowl.

5. Dressing drizzling:

Drizzle the salad with the prepared dressing.

6. Add a garnish:

Toss the salad with the roasted almond slices.

Garnish with fresh dill to add taste and a bit of green if preferred.

This Salmon and Avocado Salad is a healthy and sugar-free choice. Salmon contains omega-3 fatty acids as well as protein, while avocado contains healthful fats and fiber. The fresh veggies provide vitamins and minerals, while the dressing complements the tastes without adding sugar. As part of your sugar detox plan, enjoy this tasty and nutritious salad.

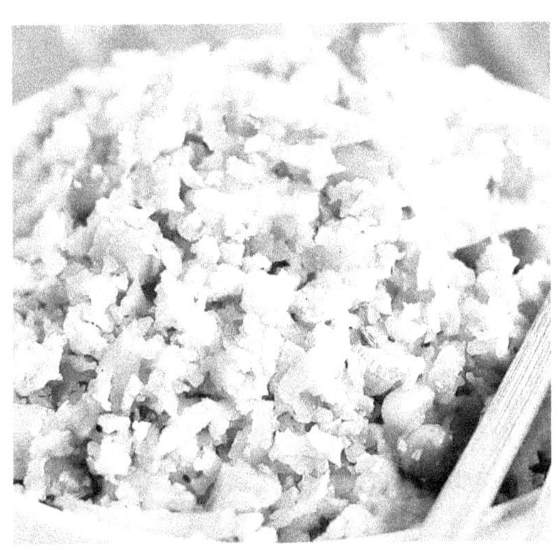

Ingredients:

1 medium head cauliflower, cut into florets

2 tbsp olive oil or coconut oil

1/2 cup carrots, chopped

1 frozen cup peas

1/2 cup red bell pepper, chopped

1/2 cup red onion, chopped

2 minced garlic cloves

2 big beaten eggs

2 tbsp low-sodium soy sauce (or sugar-free soy sauce substitute)

1/2 teaspoon ginger powder

Season with salt and black pepper to taste.

Optional garnish: chopped green onions

Instructions:

1. Gather Your Ingredients:

In a food processor, pulse the cauliflower florets until they resemble rice grains. If you don't have a food processor, you may use a grater instead.

Cut the carrots, red bell pepper, and red onion into dice.

Garlic should be minced

2. Sauté Vegetables:

Heat the coconut oil or olive oil in a large pan or wok over medium-high heat.

Combine the chopped carrots, frozen peas, diced red bell pepper, and diced red onion in a mixing bowl. Sauté for 5-7 minutes or until the veggies soften.

3. Stir in the garlic and cauliflower rice:

Sauté the minced garlic in the skillet for a further 1-2 minutes, or until aromatic.

Stir in the cauliflower rice to mix with the other veggies in the pan.

4. Prepare Cauliflower Rice:

Cook for another 5-7 minutes, stirring periodically, until the cauliflower rice is soft and slightly brown.

5. Set aside the rice:

Place the cauliflower rice on one side of the skillet and the beaten eggs on the other.

6. Scrambled eggs:

Scramble the eggs until completely cooked.

7. Mix and season:

Combine the scrambled eggs and cauliflower rice.

To taste, add low-sodium soy sauce (or a sugar-free soy sauce substitute), ground ginger, salt, and black pepper.

For taste, season with salt and pepper.

8. Garnish:

Garnish the Cauliflower Fried Rice with chopped green onions if desired.

Cauliflower Fried Rice is a low-carb and sugar-free alternative to classic fried rice. It's low in carbohydrates and high in veggies. The cauliflower rice lends a pleasing texture, and the spice adds taste without the need of additional sugars. As part of your sugar detox regimen, enjoy this tasty and healthy dinner.

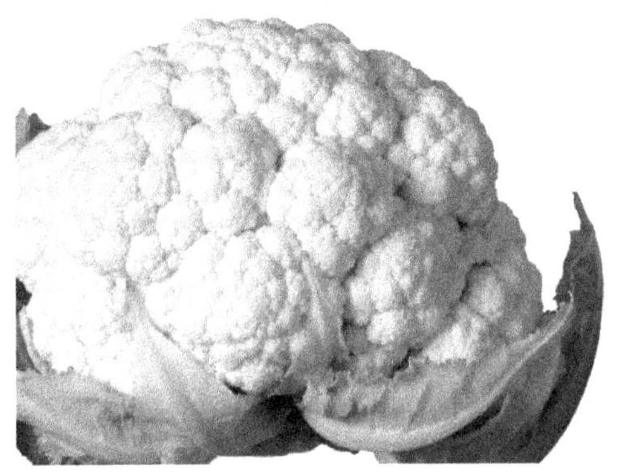

calliflower

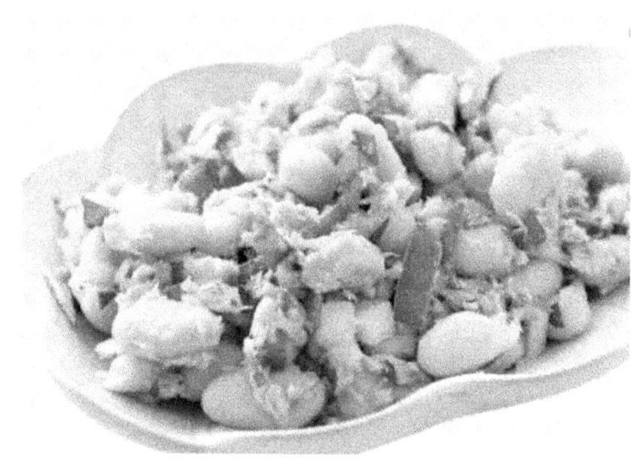

Ingredients:

2 drained cans (5 ounces each) of canned tuna

2 cans (15 oz. each) drained and washed white beans (cannellini or navy beans)

1/2 coarsely chopped red onion

1/2 cup fresh parsley, chopped

1 tablespoon extra-virgin olive oil

1 lemon juice

2 minced garlic cloves

For taste, add salt and black pepper.

Optional garnish: cherry tomatoes

Garnish with fresh basil leaves (optional).

Instructions:

1. Gather Your Ingredients:

Drain and flake the canned tuna into bite-sized pieces.

The white beans should be drained and rinsed.

Chop the red onion and fresh parsley finely.

Garlic should be minced.

2. Prepare the Dressing:

Whisk together the extra-virgin olive oil, lemon juice, minced garlic, salt, and black pepper to taste in a small bowl. Set aside the dressing.

3. Mix tuna, white beans, and vegetables:

Combine the flaked tuna, white beans, diced red onion, and fresh parsley in a large mixing basin.

4. Drizzle with dressing:

Dress the tuna and white bean combination with the dressing.

5. Toss everything together:

Toss everything together gently to cover everything with the dressing.

6. Add a garnish:

Garnish the Tuna and White Bean Salad with cherry tomatoes and fresh basil leaves, if preferred.

This Tuna and White Bean Salad is high in protein and low in sugar. White beans give fiber and a creamy texture, while tuna supplies lean protein. The fresh herbs and spicy dressing complement the tastes without adding any sweetness. As part of your sugar detox strategy, enjoy this nutritious and tasty salad.

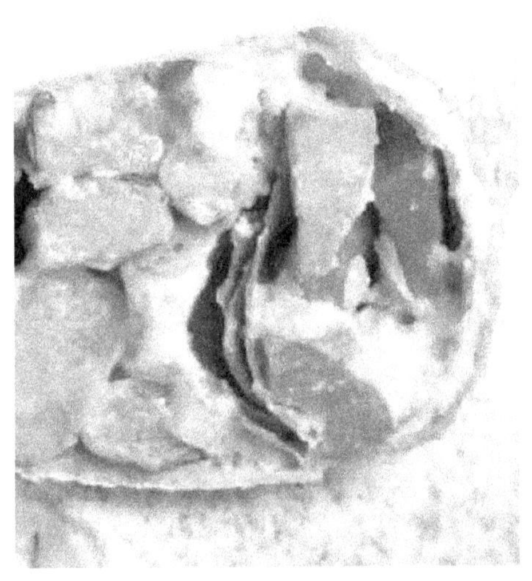

Ingredients:

To make the roasted vegetables:

2 cups sliced or halved mixed veggies, such as bell peppers, zucchini, red onion, and cherry tomatoes

2 tbsp of olive oil

1 tsp. dried oregano

Add salt and pepper to taste.

For the Finish:

1 whole-grain or whole-wheat tortilla (no added sugars preferred)

1/4 cup hummus (preferably sugar-free)

1/4 cup crumbled feta cheese (optional; substitute a dairy-free version if preferred)

Spinach leaves, fresh

Optional: sliced black olives

Fresh basil leaves for flavoring and garnishing (optional).

Instructions:

1. Gather Your Ingredients:

Cut the veggies into thin strips or half.

2. Vegetables, roasted:

Preheat the oven to 200 degrees Celsius.

Toss the mixed veggies with olive oil, dried oregano, salt, and black pepper in a mixing bowl.

Place the seasoned veggies on a baking sheet and bake for 15-20 minutes, or until soft and slightly browned.

3. Put the Wrap Together:

Place a whole-grain or whole-wheat tortilla on a clean surface.

4. Distribute Hummus:

Spread hummus evenly on the tortilla.

5. Include roasted vegetables:

Serve the hummus with the roasted vegetables on top.

6. Top with Feta Cheese:

To add flavor, sprinkle crumbled feta cheese over the vegetables.

7. Pile on the spinach and olives:

If preferred, garnish with fresh spinach leaves and sliced black olives.

8. Garnish:

Place fresh basil leaves on top of the ingredients for more flavor and garnish.

9. Wrap it up:

Fold in the edges of the tortilla carefully, then roll it up firmly to make the wrap.

10. Serve and Have Fun:

To make it simpler to handle, cut the Roasted Veggie and Hummus Wrap in half.

Serve and enjoy a delectable and sugar-free dinner.

This Roasted Veggie and Hummus Wrap is a filling and nutritious sugar-detox option. The roasted veggies offer natural sweetness as well as vitamins and minerals, while the hummus and feta cheese bring creaminess and taste. Fresh spinach and basil leaves give flavor and nutrients to the wrap without adding sweetness. As part of your sugar detox regimen, enjoy this healthful and tasty wrap.

Day 22: Baked Lemon Herb Chicken

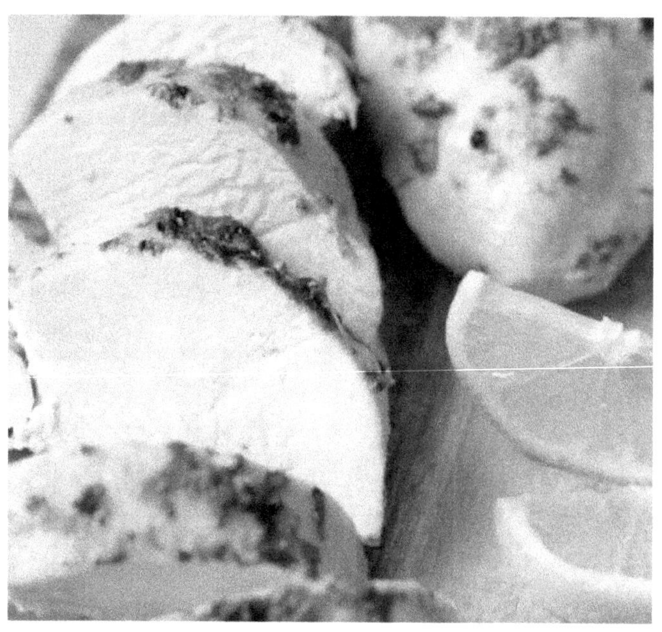

Ingredients:

4 skinless, boneless chicken breasts

2 tbsp of olive oil

1 lemon's zest

2 lemons juice

3 minced garlic cloves

1 teaspoon thyme dried

1 teaspoon rosemary dried

1 tsp. dried oregano

Add salt and black pepper to taste.

Optional garnish: lemon slices

Garnish with fresh herbs such as parsley or thyme (optional).

Instructions:

1. Gather Your Ingredients:

Preheat the oven to 190 degrees Celsius.

Squeeze the lemon and zest it.

Garlic should be minced.

2. Prepare the marinade:

Mix together the olive oil, lemon zest, lemon juice, minced garlic, dried thyme, dried rosemary, dried oregano, salt, and black pepper in a mixing bowl.

To make the marinade, mix all the ingredients together in a bowl

3. Prepare the marinade for the chicken:

Put the chicken breasts in a zip-top bag or shallow dish and set aside.

Pour the marinade over the chicken and toss to coat evenly.

Refrigerate the dish or seal the bag for at least 30 minutes to enable the flavors to infuse.

4. Cook the chicken in the oven:

Place the marinated chicken breasts on a baking pan.

Any leftover marinade should be poured over the chicken.

Bake for 25-30 minutes, or until the chicken is well cooked and an internal temperature of 165°F (74°C) is reached.

5. Decorate and serve:

Remove the Baked Lemon Herb Chicken from the oven when it is done.

For extra taste and presentation, garnish with lemon slices and fresh herbs (such as parsley or thyme).

This Baked Lemon Herb Chicken is a tasty and sugar-free option. The lemon and herb combination provides zest and perfume to the chicken without the need for additional sweeteners. As part of your sugar detox regimen, enjoy this tasty and healthful chicken dinner.

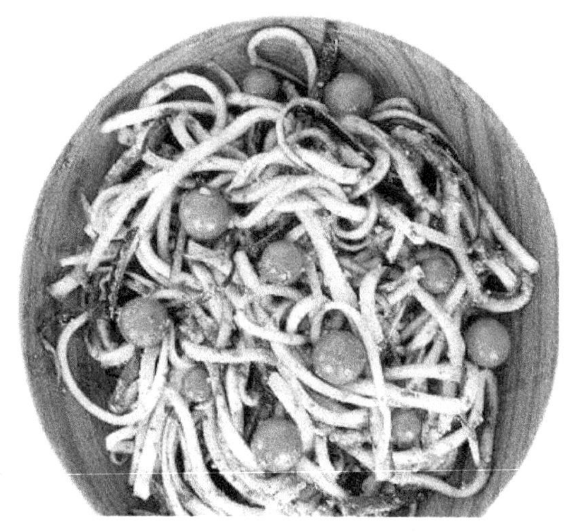

Ingredients:

To make the pesto:

2 cups basil leaves, fresh

1/2 cup pine nuts (lightly roast them for more taste)

1/2 cup grated Parmesan cheese (optional; if preferred, use a dairy-free substitute)

2 minced garlic cloves

1 tablespoon extra-virgin olive oil

1 lemon juice

Add salt and black pepper to taste.

To make the Zucchini Noodles:

4 large zucchinis

1 tablespoon extra-virgin olive oil

Add salt and black pepper to taste.

Instructions:

1. Gather Your Ingredients:

The zucchinis should be washed and dried.

If desired, lightly toast the pine nuts.

If used, grate the Parmesan cheese.

2. Prepare the Pesto:

Combine the fresh basil leaves, pine nuts, grated Parmesan cheese (if using), minced garlic, extra-virgin olive oil, lemon juice, salt, and black pepper to taste in a food processor.

Pulse the ingredients until it achieves the appropriate consistency. Depending on your preferences, you may make it smooth or somewhat lumpy.

Season with salt and pepper to taste.

3. Make the Zucchini Noodles:

Create zucchini noodles from the zucchinis using a spiralizer or a julienne peeler. You may finely julienne the zucchinis by hand if you don't have these equipment.

4. Zucchini Noodles Sauté:

Heat the oil in a big pan over medium heat.

Sauté the zucchini noodles for about 2-3 minutes, or until soft. Don't overcook them; they should still have a tiny crunch.

5. Toss with pesto:

Remove the pan from the heat and toss the sautéed zucchini noodles with the prepared pesto.Toss the noodles in the pesto until evenly covered.

6. Garnish and serve:

Serve the Zucchini Noodles with Pesto on plates.

Garnish with more pine nuts, fresh basil leaves, and a sprinkling of Parmesan cheese (or a dairy-free substitute) if preferred.

These Zucchini Noodles with Pesto are a tasty and sugar-free supper. The zucchini noodles are a low-carb, low-sugar alternative to typical pasta, and the homemade pesto is flavorful without being loaded with sugar. As part of your sugar detox strategy, enjoy this fresh and healthful dinner.

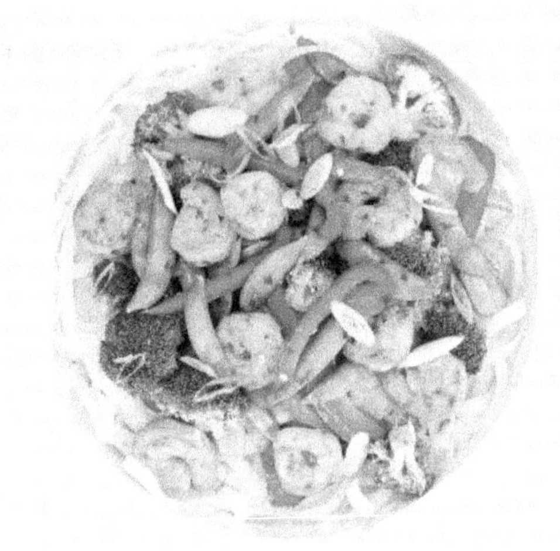

Ingredients:

To make the Stir-Fry Sauce:

3 tbsp low-sodium soy sauce (or sugar-free soy sauce substitute)

1 tablespoon vinegar (rice)

1 tablespoon honey replacement (e.g., stevia, erythritol, or your preferred sugar-free sweetener)

1 tbsp sesame oil

1 tsp cornstarch or arrowroot powder (for thickening)

1/2 teaspoon red pepper flakes (modify to spice preference.)

To make the stir-fry:

1 pound big peeled and deveined shrimp

2 tbsp of olive oil

3 garlic cloves, minced 1 inch fresh ginger, minced 1 red bell pepper, sliced 1 yellow bell pepper, sliced

1 cup florets broccoli

1 pound snap peas

Season with salt and black pepper to taste.

Serve with brown rice or cauliflower rice cooked.

Instructions:

1. Gather Your Ingredients:

In a small mixing bowl, combine the stir-fry sauce ingredients: low-sodium soy sauce, rice vinegar, honey alternative, sesame oil, cornstarch (or arrowroot powder), and red pepper flakes.

Peel and devein the shrimp before patting them dry.

Garlic and ginger should be minced.

Cut the red and yellow bell peppers into slices.

Make florets out of the broccoli.

Trim the snap peas' ends.

2. Prepare the Shrimp:

In a large pan or wok, heat 1 tablespoon olive oil over medium-high heat.

Cook for approximately 1-2 minutes on each side, or until the shrimp turn pink and opaque. Set the shrimp aside after removing them from the skillet.

3. Cook Aromatics and Vegetables:

In the same skillet, add the remaining 1 tablespoon olive oil to the same skillet.

Sauté the minced garlic and ginger for 30 seconds, or until fragrant.

Combine the sliced bell peppers, broccoli, and snap peas in a mixing bowl. Cook, stirring occasionally, for 3-4 minutes, or until the veggies are tender-crisp.

4. Mix and thicken:

Add the cooked shrimp back to the skillet.

Serve the shrimp and veggies with the stir-fry sauce.

Stir everything together and let aside for a minute or two to thicken the sauce.

5. Seasoning and serving:

Season to taste with salt and black pepper.

Over cooked brown rice or cauliflower rice, serve the Spicy Shrimp Stir-Fry.

This Spicy Shrimp Stir-Fry is a tasty and sugar-free choice. The stir-fry sauce has a sweet, savory, and spicy taste profile with no added sweeteners. It's a tasty and low-carb supper alternative for your sugar detox. Enjoy!

Day 25: Stuffed Bell Peppers

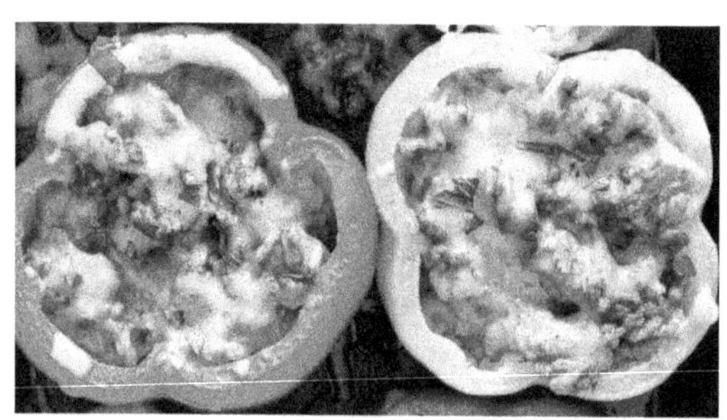

Ingredients:

For the Stuffed Bell Peppers, use the following ingredients:

4 big colored bell peppers

1 pound ground turkey or chicken, lean

1/2 cup washed and cooked quinoa, according to package directions

1 cup chopped tomatoes (fresh or canned)

1/2 cup onion, chopped

1/2 cup zucchini, diced

2 minced garlic cloves

1 tsp. dried oregano

a half teaspoon dried basil

Topping: salt and black pepper to taste

1/2 cup grated Parmesan cheese (optional; if preferred, use a dairy-free substitute)

Garnish with fresh parsley or basil (optional).

Instructions:

1. Gather Your Ingredients:

Preheat the oven to 190 degrees Celsius.

Remove the tops of the bell peppers, as well as any membranes and seeds. Place aside.

Follow the package directions for cooking the quinoa.

Tomatoes, onion, zucchini, and garlic should all be diced.

Brown the ground beef:

Cook the ground turkey or chicken in a large pan over medium heat until no longer pink. Remove any extra fat.

3. Seasonings and vegetables:

Add the diced tomatoes, onion, zucchini, and minced garlic to the cooked ground beef.

Stir in the cooked quinoa, oregano, basil, salt, and black pepper to taste.

Cook, stirring occasionally, until the veggies are soft.

4. Fill the bell peppers with:

Stuff the prepped bell peppers with the meat and quinoa mixture with care.

5. Optional cheese topping:

If desired, top the filled bell peppers with grated Parmesan cheese.

6. Bake:

Cover the filled bell peppers in a baking dish with foil.

Bake the bell peppers for 25-30 minutes, or until soft.

7. Decorate and serve:

Remove the foil and, if desired, sprinkle with fresh parsley or basil for additional taste and color.

These Stuffed Bell Peppers are a nutritious and sugar-free lunch alternative. A balanced and healthy dish is created by combining lean ground beef, quinoa, and a variety of veggies. The extra Parmesan cheese offers a taste boost, but you can leave it out for a dairy-free version. As part of your sugar detox regimen, enjoy this tasty and filling lunch.

Day 26: Cilantro Lime Grilled Salmon

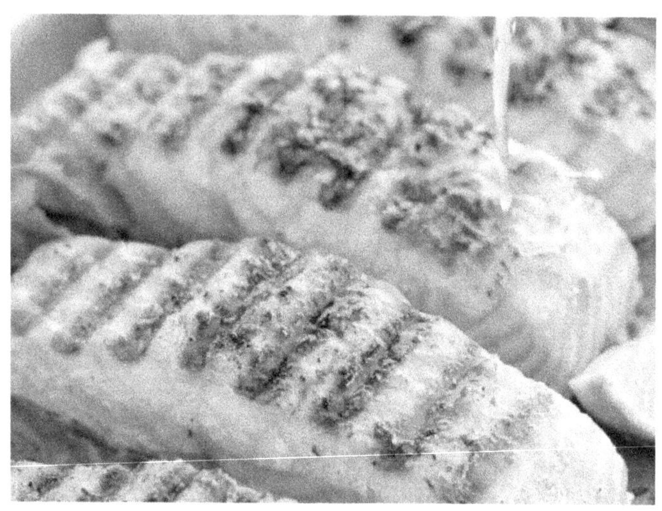

Ingredients:

4 skin-on or skinless salmon fillets (6-8 ounces each)

1/4 cup chopped fresh cilantro

2 limes, zest and juice

2 minced garlic cloves

2 tbsp of olive oil

1 teaspoon cumin powder

Add salt and black pepper to taste.

Optional garnish: lime wedges

Optional extra cilantro for garnish

Instructions:

1. Gather Your Ingredients:

Preheat the grill to medium-high.

2. Prepare the marinade:

Combine the cilantro, lime zest, lime juice, minced garlic, olive oil, ground cumin, salt, and black pepper to taste in a small bowl.

3. Marinate the salmon as follows:

Fill a plate or a reseal- able plastic bag halfway with salmon fillets.

Pour the cilantro lime marinade over the salmon and coat each fillet evenly. Marinate for 15 minutes to 30 minutes.

4. Cook the salmon on the grill:

Lightly oil the grill grates to prevent sticking.

Grill the salmon fillets, skin side down, or immediately on the grill grates if skinless.

Grill the salmon for approximately 4-5 minutes each side, or until it's cooked through and flakes easily with a fork. If there is skin, it should be crispy.

5. Decorate and serve:

Take the cooked salmon off the grill.

If preferred, garnish with lime wedges and additional cilantro.

Serve the Cilantro Lime Grilled Salmon at room temperature.

This Cilantro Lime Grilled Salmon is a tasty and sugar-free choice. The tangy cilantro and lime marinade adds a blast of fresh flavor to the salmon without adding sweetness. It's a nutritious and tasty dish to eat as part of your sugar detox regimen.

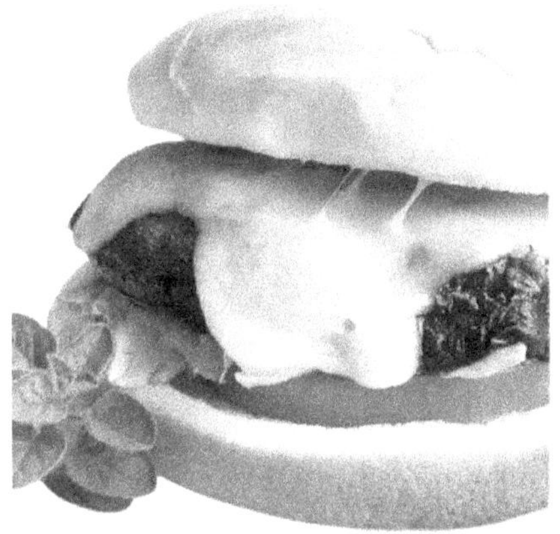

Ingredients:

To make the Mushroom Caps:

4 big portobello mushroom tops, removed stems

2 tbsp of olive oil

2 minced garlic cloves

2 tbsp balsamic vinegar

Add salt and black pepper to taste.

Toppings for the Burger:

4 whole-grain or whole-wheat burger buns (no added sugars preferred)

4 slices cheese of your choice (optional, substitute dairy-free if preferred)

Tomato slices

Red onion, thinly sliced

Lettuce or spinach leaves, fresh

Optional: Dijon mustard or sugar-free ketchup

Optional pickles

Instructions:

1. Gather Your Ingredients:

Preheat the grill or grill pan to medium-high.

2. Wash and Marinate Mushroom Caps:

Brush away any dirt from the portobello mushroom tops.

Whisk together the olive oil, minced garlic, balsamic vinegar, salt, and black pepper in a mixing bowl.

Brush the marinade on both sides of the mushroom caps.

3. Cook the Mushrooms:

Place the marinated mushroom caps on the grill or grill pan that has been warmed.

Grill for approximately 4-5 minutes each side, or until soft and grill marks form. Because the mushrooms will shed moisture, spray them with any residual marinade while cooking.

4. Optional: Add cheese:

Place a piece of cheese on each mushroom cap during the last minute of grilling to enable it to melt.

5. Make the Burgers:

Grill the burger buns for about a minute, or until they are mildly crispy.

On the bottom half of each bun, place a grilled portobello mushroom cap.

Top with sliced tomatoes, red onion, fresh lettuce or spinach leaves, and your favorite condiments or pickles.

6. Serve and Have Fun:

To finish your Portobello Mushroom Burgers, place the top half of the burger buns on each mushroom.

Serve and enjoy your delectable and sugar-free burger.

These Portobello Mushroom Burgers are a delicious and nutritious alternative to regular burgers. The marinated and grilled portobello mushrooms give a robust, umami-rich taste without the use of added sweeteners. As part of your sugar detox strategy, choose your toppings and enjoy this nutritious burger.

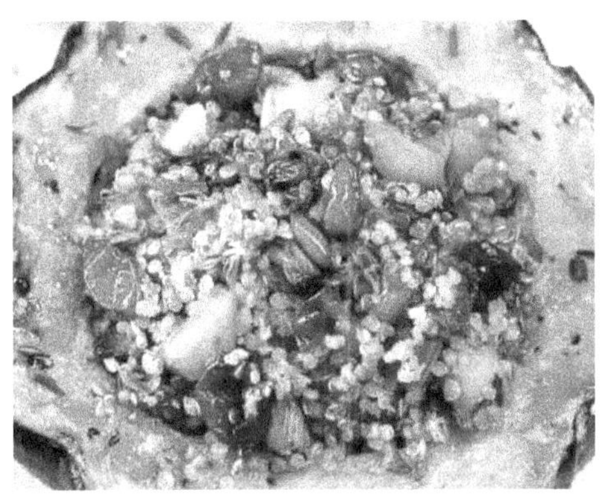

Ingredients:

2 acorn squash, peeled and halved

1 cup washed and cooked quinoa, according to package directions

2 cups water or vegetable broth

1 tablespoon extra virgin olive oil

1/2 cup chopped red bell pepper 1/2 cup diced onion

1/2 cup zucchini, diced

2 minced garlic cloves

1 teaspoon cumin powder

1/2 teaspoon coriander powder

Add salt and black pepper to taste.

Garnish with chopped fresh parsley or cilantro (optional).

Instructions:

1. Gather Your Ingredients:

Preheat the oven to 190 degrees Celsius.

2. Squash Preparation:

Scoop off the seeds and threads from the acorn squash by cutting it in half. If necessary, cut a little slice off the bottoms to help them sit flat in the baking dish.

3. Bake the Squash:

Place the acorn squash halves cut-side down in a baking dish and cover with approximately 1/2 inch of water.

Bake for 30-35 minutes, or until the squash is soft and a fork can easily be inserted.

4. Prepare Quinoa:

While the squash bakes, rinse and boil the quinoa according to package directions, adding flavor with vegetable broth or water.

5. Make the Filling:

Heat the olive oil in a pan over medium heat.

Toss in the onion, red bell pepper, and zucchini. Fry the veggies for 5 minutes, or until tender.

6. Seasonings:

Mix in the minced garlic, cumin, coriander, salt, and black pepper. Sauté for another 2 minutes, or until aromatic.

7. Mix Quinoa and Vegetables:

Combine the sautéed veggie combination and cooked quinoa.

8. Fill the Squash:

Remove the acorn squash halves from the oven when they are tender.

Flip them over carefully so that the cut-side is up.

Fill each squash half halfway with the quinoa-vegetable mixture.

9. Garnish:

For extra flavor and appearance, garnish the Quinoa-Stuffed Acorn Squash with chopped fresh parsley or cilantro.

These Quinoa-Stuffed Acorn Squash Halves are a filling and sugar-free dinner. Quinoa, sautéed veggies, and acorn squash give a nice blend of tastes and textures without any added sweeteners. As part of your sugar detox regimen, enjoy this healthful and tasty dinner.

Chapter 3

SNACKS AND DESSERTS

Sugar-Free Snack Ideas

Sugar-free snacks may be a tasty and fulfilling addition to any sugar detox regimen. Here are some sugar-free snack suggestions:

Fresh fruits: While certain fruits contain natural sugars, they can be included in a sugar detox regimen. Choose low-sugar foods such as berries (strawberries, blueberries, and raspberries), kiwi, and watermelon. These fruits are high in antioxidants, fiber, and vitamins.

Greek Yogurt with Berries: Choose plain Greek yogurt, which has less sugar than flavored varieties. For a naturally sweet and fulfilling snack, top it with fresh or frozen berries.

Raw Nuts: Almonds, walnuts, and cashews are excellent snack foods. They are packed in healthy fats and protein, which can help you feel fuller for longer. Always be aware that nuts are high in calories.

Hummus with Veggies: Dip fresh vegetable sticks in sugar-free hummus, such as carrots, celery, cucumber, and bell peppers. It's a fiber-rich, crispy and flavorful snack.

Hard-Boiled Eggs: Hard-boiled eggs are a high-protein food that can help you maintain your energy levels. To enhance flavor, season with a touch of salt and black pepper.

Cottage Cheese: Use plain, unsweetened cottage cheese and season with olive oil, fresh herbs, salt, and black pepper. It's a high-protein option.

Mozzarella and Cherry Tomatoes: Serve small mozzarella cheese balls with cherry tomatoes and fresh basil leaves. Drizzle with olive oil and balsamic vinegar, preferably one without added sugars.

Natural Almond or Peanut Butter and Celery:
Spread natural almond or peanut butter on celery
sticks. It's a delicious blend of crunchy and creamy
with no added sugars.

Guacamole Rice Cakes: Serve whole-grain rice
cakes with homemade guacamole (avocado, lime
juice, salt, and pepper). It's a crunchy and filling
snack.

When selecting packaged snacks, don't forget to
read the labels to make sure they are actually sugar-
free. When possible, choose whole, unprocessed
foods because they are less likely to include sugars
that are hidden. You can stick to your sugar detox
plan and maintain your energy levels with the
support of these sugar-free snacks.

Desserts are a great way to satisfy your sweet tooth while staying on track with your sugar detox plan. Natural, sugar-free sweeteners and whole ingredients are used to make these desserts. Here are some delicious sugar detox dessert recipes:

Fruit Salad: Make a colorful fruit salad with berries, citrus fruits, and melon. Without adding sugar, a squeeze of fresh lemon or lime juice can enhance the flavors.

Chia Seed Pudding: Use unsweetened almond milk or coconut milk to make chia seed pudding. Sweeten with a sugar-free sweetener such as stevia or monk fruit, and top with fresh berries for natural sweetness.

Dark Chocolate: As a treat, select high-quality dark chocolate (70% cocoa or higher). It is lower in sugar than milk chocolate and higher in antioxidants.

Baked Apples: Peel and slice the apples, then sprinkle with cinnamon and bake until tender. Warm, spiced apples make a filling dessert with no added sugars.

Greek yoghurt parfait: Layer plain Greek yogurt with fresh berries and a sprinkle of chopped nuts to make a parfait. To add sweetness, drizzle a small amount of honey or a sugar-free sweetener on top.

Coconut Macaroons: Unsweetened shredded coconut and egg whites are used to make coconut macaroons. Bake until golden brown and sweetened with a sugar-free sweetener.

Frozen Banana "Ice Cream": To make a creamy, ice cream-like treat, combine frozen bananas with a splash of unsweetened almond milk and a dash of vanilla extract.

Avocado Chocolate Mousse: To make a rich and creamy chocolate mousse, combine ripe avocados, cocoa powder, a sugar-free sweetener, and a dash of vanilla extract.

Berries with Whipped Coconut Cream: Drizzle whipped coconut cream over a bowl of mixed berries. Sweeten the cream with a sugar-free sweetener and a few drops of vanilla extract.

Day 29: Chocolate Avocado Mousse

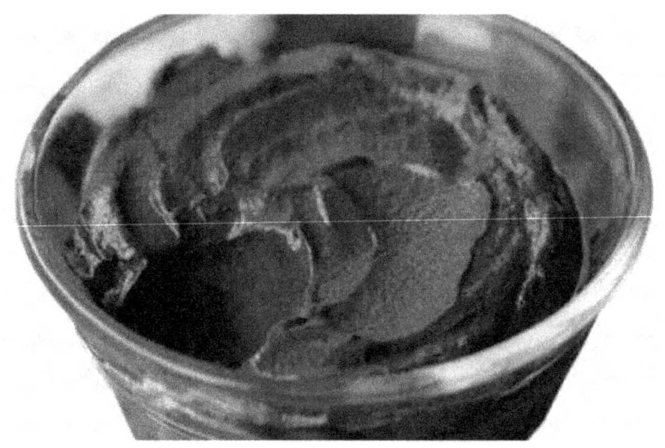

Ingredients:

2 peeled and pitted ripe avocados

1/4 cup cocoa powder, unsweetened

1/4 cup unsweetened almond milk (or your favorite unsweetened milk)

3-4 tablespoons sugar-free sweetener (stevia, erythritol, monk fruit, or to taste) a tsp vanilla extract

a grain of salt

Optional Extras:

Berries, fresh

Chopped nuts (almonds, walnuts, etc.)

Shredded unsweetened coconut

garnished with mint leaves

Instructions:

1. Gather Your Ingredients:

Check the avocados for ripeness and remove the pits.

2. Whisk together the avocado mixture:

Combine the ripe avocados, unsweetened cocoa powder, unsweetened almond milk, sugar-free sweetener, vanilla extract, and a pinch of salt in a food processor or blender.

3. Puree until smooth:

Blend the mixture until it is creamy and all of the ingredients are well combined. Adjust the sweetness to your liking by adding more sweetener if necessary or removing from it.

4. Chill:

Place the chocolate avocado mousse in a bowl or individual serving dishes and serve.

Cover and place in the refrigerator for at least 30 minutes to chill and set.

5. Serve and Garnish:

Garnish with fresh berries, chopped nuts, unsweetened shredded coconut, or a sprig of mint leaves when ready to serve.

This Chocolate Avocado Mousse is a decadent and creamy sugar-free dessert. It's a healthier alternative to traditional chocolate mousse thanks to the natural sweetness of ripe avocados and sugar-free sweetener. As part of your sugar detox, enjoy this guilt-free treat.

Day 30: Mixed Berry Chia Seed Popsicles

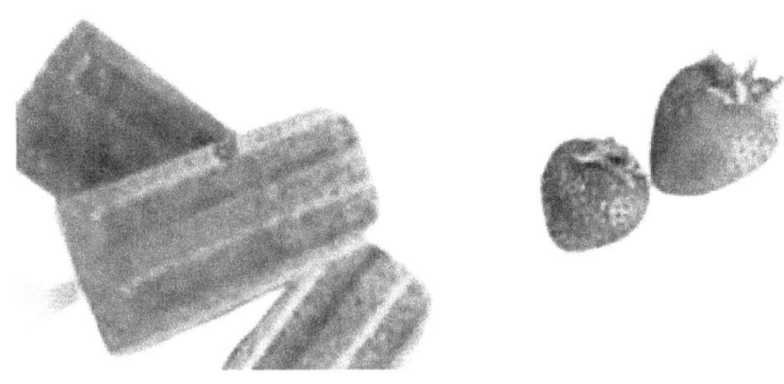

Ingredients:

2 cup berry mixture (strawberries, blueberries, raspberries, and blackberries)

2 tbsp of chia seeds

1/4 cup unsweetened almond milk (or your favorite unsweetened milk)

2-3 tbsp sugar-free sweetener of choice (stevia, erythritol, or to taste)

a tsp vanilla extract

Instructions:

1. Gather Your Ingredients:

Remove any stems from the mixed berries and rinse them.

2. Combine the Berry Mixture:

Combine the mixed berries, unsweetened almond milk, sugar-free sweetener, and vanilla extract in a blender or food processor.

Blend the mixture until it is smooth and well combined. Adjust the sweetness until your desired is met.

3. Stir in the Chia Seeds:

Add the chia seeds to the berry mixture in a mixing bowl. Mix well to distribute the chia seeds evenly throughout the mixture.

4. Fill Popsicle Molds:

Fill Popsicle molds halfway with the berry chia seed mixture, leaving a little space at the top for expansion.

Fill each mold with popsicle sticks.

5. Freeze:

Put the Popsicle molds in the freezer for at least 4-6 hours, or until they are completely solid.

6. Remove from the mold and enjoy:

Run warm water over the bottom of the molds to loosen them before removing the popsicles.

Serve your Mixed Berry Chia Seed Popsicles as a refreshing and sugar-free frozen treat.

These Mixed Berry Chia Seed Popsicles are a delicious way to enjoy a sweet, refreshing dessert while adhering to your sugar detox plan. Chia seeds provide fiber and omega-3 fatty acids, making these popsicles a healthy option. On a hot day, they're a guilt-free treat!

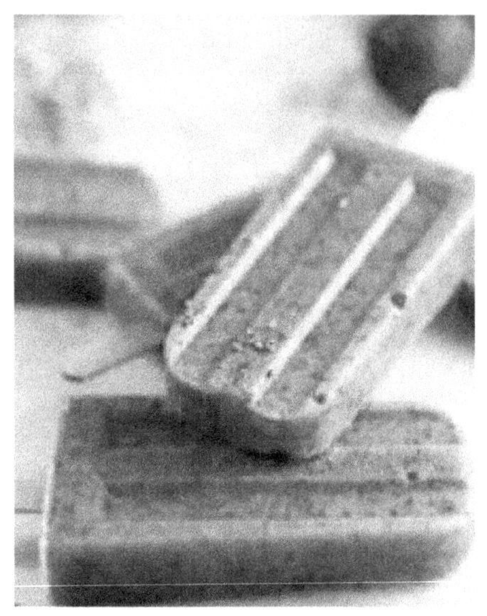

Chapter 4:

Sugar detox recipes

Breakfast recipes:

 ➢ Overnight Oats:

Ingredients:

1/2 cup certified sugar-free old-fashioned rolled oats

1/2 cup unsweetened almond milk (or your favorite unsweetened milk)

1/4 cup plain (unsweetened) Greek yogurt

a half teaspoon of vanilla extract

Optional: 1/2 teaspoon cinnamon

Toppings: fresh berries or sliced fruit (strawberries, blueberries, etc.)

For garnish, use chopped nuts or seeds (such as almonds or chia seeds).

Instructions:

1. Prepare the Base:

Combine the rolled oats, unsweetened almond milk, plain Greek yogurt, vanilla extract, and cinnamon (if using) in a jar or container with a lid.

2. Thoroughly mix:

Stir the ingredients together until well combined. Ensure that the oats are completely submerged in the liquid.

3. Store in the refrigerator overnight:

Refrigerate the jar or container overnight or for at least 4 hours after sealing it with a lid. This allows the oats to absorb and soften the liquid.

4. Optional toppings:

Bring out the oats from the fridge the next morning.

Overnight oats can be topped with fresh berries or sliced fruit of your choice. For added texture and flavor, add chopped nuts or seeds.

5. Enjoy:

After giving it a good stir to incorporate the toppings, your Sugar Detox-friendly Overnight Oats are ready to eat.

> Scrambled Eggs with Sautéed Spinach and Mushrooms

Ingredients:

Two large eggs

1 cup washed and chopped fresh spinach

1/2 cup mushrooms, sliced

1/4 cup chopped onions

1 minced garlic clove

1 tablespoon of olive oil

Add salt and pepper to taste.

Garnish with fresh herbs (e.g., parsley or chives) if desired.

Instructions:

1. Gather Your Ingredients:

Fresh spinach should be washed and chopped.

Cut the mushrooms into slices, dice the onions, and mince the garlic.

Set aside the eggs after they have been beaten.

2. Cook the Vegetables:

In a nonstick skillet over medium heat, heat the olive oil.

Sauté the diced onions and sliced mushrooms in the skillet for 3-4 minutes, or until they soften and brown.

3. Stir in the spinach and garlic:

To the skillet, add the chopped spinach and minced garlic.

Continue to cook for another 1-2 minutes, or until the spinach wilts and the garlic becomes fragrant.

Add salt and pepper to the vegetable to taste.

4. Make the scrambled eggs:

Arrange the sautéed vegetables on one side of the skillet.

Pour the beaten eggs into the skillet's empty side.

Allow the eggs to cook for a moment before gently stirring and scrambling them until they reach the desired level of doneness.

5. Garnish and serve:

Transfer the entire mixture to a plate once the eggs are done.

Garnish with fresh herbs such as parsley or chives if desired.

> ➤ Crustless Egg Muffin

Ingredients:

1 large egg

1/4 cup diced bell peppers (any color)

1/4 cup diced spinach or kale

1 tablespoon diced onions

1 tablespoon diced tomatoes

Salt and pepper to taste

Cooking spray or a touch of olive oil for greasing the muffin tin

Instructions:

1. Prepare Your Ingredients:

Dice the bell peppers, spinach or kale, onions, and tomatoes.

2. Preheat the Oven:

Preheat your oven to 350°F (175°C).

3. Butter the Muffin Tin:

Grease a standard-sized muffin tin lightly with cooking spray or olive oil.

4. Arrange the Vegetables:

Place the diced bell peppers, spinach or kale, onions, and tomatoes in one of the muffin cups.

5. Crack the egg:

In the same muffin cup, crack the egg over the vegetables.

6: Season:

Season the egg and vegetable mixture with salt and pepper to taste.

7. Bake:

Place the muffin tin in a preheated oven for 15-20 minutes, or until the egg is set and cooked to your liking.

8. Serve:

Remove the crustless egg muffin from the muffin tin once it has finished cooking.

Allow it to cool for a moment before serving.

Ingredients:

1 bunch washed and trimmed broccoli rabe

two large eggs

2 slices whole-grain or sprouted-grain bread (with no added sugars)

2 minced garlic cloves

1 tablespoon extra virgin olive oil

Optional red pepper flakes (for extra heat)

Season with salt and pepper to taste.

Parmesan cheese, grated (optional, for garnish)

Instructions:

1. Begin by preparing the broccoli rabe:

Trim any tough stems from the broccoli rabe. Divide it into bite-size pieces.

2. Prepare the Broccoli Rabe:

In a large pot, water should be brought to a boil.

Blanch the broccoli rabe for about 2 minutes in boiling water. Set aside after draining.

3. Garlic and Broccoli Rabe Sauté:

Warm the olive oil in a skillet over medium heat.

Sauté the minced garlic for 30 seconds, or until fragrant.

Sauté the blanched broccoli rabe in the skillet for another 2-3 minutes, or until tender and slightly crispy.

Season with salt, pepper, and red pepper flakes to taste.

4. Eggs poached or fried:

While the broccoli rabe is cooking, poach or fry the eggs to your liking.

5. Toasted Bread:

Toast the whole-grain or sprouted-grain bread slices until golden brown.

6. Make the Toast:

Place the toasted bread slices on top of the sautéed broccoli rabe.

Top with a poached or fried egg.

7. Decorate and serve:

Season with red pepper flakes, grated Parmesan cheese (if using), and salt and pepper to taste.

> ➢ **Breakfast tortilla**

Ingredients:

Two large eggs

1 whole-grain or sprouted-grain tortilla (choose one without added sugars)

1/4 cup diced (any color) bell peppers

1/4 cup chopped onions

1/4 cup diced tomatoes

1/4 cup chopped spinach

1/4 cup shredded cheese (optional)

1 tablespoon of olive oil

Season with salt and pepper to taste.

Fresh herbs (e.g., chives or parsley) for garnish (optional)

Instructions:

1. Gather Your Ingredients:

Chop the spinach and dice the bell peppers, onions, and tomatoes

Whisk the eggs together in a bowl .

2. Cook the Vegetables:

In a nonstick skillet over medium heat, heat the olive oil.

Sauté the diced onions and bell peppers in the skillet for 3-4 minutes, or until they begin to soften.

3. Toss in the tomatoes and spinach:

To the skillet, add the diced tomatoes and spinach.

Cook for another 2 minutes, or until the spinach wilts.

4. Make the scrambled eggs:

Arrange the sautéed vegetables on one side of the skillet.

Pour the beaten eggs into the skillet's empty side.

Allow the eggs to cook for a moment before gently stirring and scrambling them to the desired level of doneness.

5. Preheat the Tortilla:

While the eggs cook, warm the whole-grain or sprouted-grain tortilla in a dry skillet for 30 seconds on each side, or until it's warm and slightly crispy.

6. Put together the Breakfast Tortilla:

Fill the center of the warm tortilla with scrambled eggs.

If using cheese, sprinkle it on top of the eggs.

7. Decorate and serve:

If desired, garnish with fresh herbs.

Fold or roll the tortilla in half like a burrito.

Lunch recipes:

➢ Detox Lentil Soup:

Ingredients:

1 cup rinsed and drained dried green or brown lentils

1 large chopped onion

2 diced carrots

2 celery stalks, diced 3 garlic cloves, minced 1 can (14 oz) tomatoes, diced (no sugar added)

6 cups vegetable broth (low sodium, no sugar added)

2 tbsp. olive oil

1 teaspoon cumin powder

1 teaspoon turmeric powder

1/2 teaspoon coriander powder

Add salt and black pepper to taste.

Garnish with fresh parsley or cilantro (optional).

Instructions:

1. Make the Lentils:

Drain and rinse the dried lentils.

2. Cook the Aromatics:

Warm the olive oil in a large soup pot over medium heat.

Mix in the onion, carrots, and celery.

Sauté the vegetables for 5-7 minutes, or until softened and the onions are translucent.

3. Season with spices and garlic:

Mix in the minced garlic, ground cumin, turmeric, and coriander.

Continue to cook for another minute, or until fragrant.

4. Stir in the lentils, tomatoes, and broth:

Pour in the rinsed lentils, diced tomatoes, and vegetable broth.

To combine, stir everything together.

5. Simmering:

Bring the mixture to a boil, then turn it down low.

Cook, covered, for 25-30 minutes, or until the lentils are tender.

6 Season:

Add salt and black pepper to the soup to taste. Adjust the seasoning as desired.

7. Serve:

Pour the soup into individual bowls.

If desired, garnish with fresh parsley or cilantro.

Ingredients:

To make the grilled chicken:

2 skinless, boneless chicken breasts

1 tablespoon extra virgin olive oil

1 paprika teaspoon

a half teaspoon cumin

Season with salt and pepper to taste.

To make the lettuce wraps:

Large lettuce leaves (iceberg or butter lettuce, for example)

1 cup tomato dice

1/2 cup cucumbers, diced

1/4 cup red onion, diced

1/4 cup fresh cilantro or mint, chopped

1/4 cup plain (unsweetened) Greek yogurt

One lime juice

Optional hot sauce or sriracha (for extra heat)

Instructions:

1. Cook the grilled chicken:

Preheat the grill to medium-high temperature.

In a small mixing bowl, combine the olive oil, paprika, cumin, salt, and pepper.

Brush this mixture over the chicken breasts.

2. Cook the chicken on the grill:

Grill the chicken breasts for 6-8 minutes per side, or until cooked through and grill marks appear.

Remove from the grill and set aside for a few minutes before slicing the chicken into thin strips.

3. Assemble the lettuce wraps as follows:

Place a few strips of grilled chicken in the center of a large lettuce leaf.

Toss in diced tomatoes, cucumbers, red onions, and cilantro or mint to taste.

Drizzle some plain Greek yogurt on top of the fillings.

For extra flavor, squeeze fresh lime juice over the top.

Drizzle with hot sauce or sriracha if you like it spicy.

4. Wrap and Serve:

Fold the lettuce leaf around the fillings like a taco or burrito.

Secure with toothpicks if needed.

Repeat with the remaining lettuce leaves and fillings.

> Greek salad with grilled shrimp

Ingredients:

To make the grilled chicken:

2 skinless, boneless chicken breasts

1 tablespoon extra virgin olive oil

1 paprika teaspoon

a half teaspoon cumin

Season with salt and pepper to taste.

To make the lettuce wraps:

Large lettuce leaves (iceberg or butter lettuce, for example)

1 cup tomato dice

1/2 cup cucumbers, diced

1/4 cup red onion, diced

1/4 cup fresh cilantro or mint, chopped

1/4 cup plain (unsweetened) Greek yogurt

One lime juice

Optional hot sauce or sriracha (for extra heat)

Instructions:

1. Cook the grilled chicken:

Preheat the grill to medium-high temperature.

In a small mixing bowl, combine the olive oil, paprika, cumin, salt, and pepper.

Brush this mixture over the chicken breasts.

2. Cook the chicken on the grill:

Grill the chicken breasts for 6-8 minutes per side, or until cooked through and grill marks appear.

Remove from the grill and set aside for a few minutes before slicing the chicken into thin strips.

3. Assemble the lettuce wraps as follows:

Place a few strips of grilled chicken in the center of a large lettuce leaf.

Toss in diced tomatoes, cucumbers, red onions, and cilantro or mint to taste.

Drizzle some plain Greek yogurt on top of the fillings.

For extra flavor, squeeze fresh lime juice over the top.

Drizzle with hot sauce or sriracha if you like it spicy.

4. Wrap and Serve:

Like a taco or burrito, wrap the lettuce leaf around the fillings.

If necessary, secure with toothpicks.

Rep with the rest of the lettuce leaves and fillings.

> **Spinach and feta stuffed chicken breast**

Ingredients:

To make the Stuffed Chicken:

2 skinless, boneless chicken breasts

1 cup chopped fresh spinach

1/2 cup crumbled feta cheese (use sparingly)

2 minced garlic cloves

1 tablespoon extra virgin olive oil

Season with salt and pepper to taste.

Securing with toothpicks or kitchen twine

To prepare the Lemon Garlic Sauce:

1 lemon juice

2 tbsp of olive oil

2 minced garlic cloves

1 tsp. dried oregano

Season with salt and pepper to taste.

Instructions:

1. Make the Spinach-Feta Stuffing:

1 tablespoon olive oil, heated in a skillet over medium heat.

Mix in the minced garlic and spinach.

Cook for 3 minutes until the spinach has wilted.

Bring down from the heat and set aside to cool slightly.

Combine the sautéed spinach, crumbled feta cheese, salt, and pepper in a mixing bowl.

2. Chicken Preparation:

Preheat the oven to 190 degrees Celsius.

Butterfly the chicken breasts by cutting a horizontal line through the thickest part and leaving one edge intact to form a pocket.

3. Fill the Chicken:

Stuff each chicken breast with the spinach and feta mixture with care.

To keep the stuffing in place, secure the open ends with toothpicks or kitchen twine.

4. Seasoning and Searing:

Sprinkle salt and pepper over the stuffed chicken breasts.

Heat some olive oil in an ovenproof skillet over medium-high heat.

Sear the stuffed chicken breasts for about 2-3 minutes on each side, or until they develop a golden brown crust.

5. Bake:

Place the skillet in a preheated oven.

Bake for 20-25 minutes, or until the chicken is thoroughly cooked and no longer pink on the inside.

6. Prepare the Lemon Garlic Sauce:

While the chicken is baking, make the sauce in a small bowl by combining the lemon juice, olive oil, minced garlic, dried oregano, salt, and pepper.

7. Serve:

Remove the toothpicks or twine once the chicken is cooked.

Over the stuffed chicken breasts, drizzle the lemon garlic sauce.

Ingredients:

2 canned tuna cans (5 oz each) in water, drained

1/2 cup celery, diced

1/4 cup red onion, diced

1/4 cup diced pickles (dill or sugar-free pickles)

1/4 cup plain (unsweetened) Greek yogurt

1 tbsp. Dijon mustard

1 tablespoon freshly squeezed lemon juice

Season with salt and pepper to taste.

Garnish with fresh parsley or chives (optional).

Instructions:

1. Make the Tuna:

Open and drain the tuna can.

2. Combine the following ingredients:

Combine the drained tuna, diced celery, diced red onion, and diced pickles in a large mixing bowl.

3. Prepare the Dressing:

Whisk together the plain Greek yogurt, Dijon mustard, and fresh lemon juice in a separate bowl.

4. Toss and combine:

Dress the tuna and vegetable mixture with the dressing.

Toss all of the ingredients together gently until evenly coated.

5. The season:

Season with salt and pepper to taste.

6. Add a garnish:

Garnish with fresh parsley or chives to add color and flavor if desired.

7. Serve:

Serve the tuna salad on a bed of lettuce, in a whole-grain wrap, or with whole-grain crackers as a sandwich filling.

Dinner recipes:

> Carrot meatball with mint cauliflower rice

Ingredients:

To make the Carrot Meatballs:

2 cups carrots, grated

1 cup ground chicken or turkey, lean

1 tablespoon almond flour

1/4 cup grated Parmesan cheese (optional; use sparingly)

1/4 cup chopped onions

2 minced garlic cloves

1 egg

1 teaspoon cumin powder

paprika, 1/2 teaspoon

Season with salt and pepper to taste.

Cooking with olive oil

To prepare the Mint Cauliflower Rice:

1 small cauliflower head, cut into florets

2 tbsp of olive oil

1/4 cup fresh mint leaves, chopped 1 lemon juice

Add salt and pepper to taste.

Instructions:

<u>To make the Carrot Meatballs:</u>

1. Carrot Preparation:

Using a box grater or food processor, grate the carrots.

Squeeze out any excess moisture from the grated carrots using a clean kitchen towel.

2. Combine the following ingredients for the meatballs:

Mix together the grated carrots, ground chicken or turkey, almond flour, grated Parmesan cheese (if using), diced onions, minced garlic, egg, ground cumin, paprika, salt, and pepper in a large mixing bowl.

Combine all of the ingredients in a mixing bowl.

3. Shape the Meatballs:

Form the mixture into meatballs of your choice.

4. Prepare the Meatballs:

In a large skillet over medium-high heat, heat some olive oil.

Cook the meatballs in the skillet for 4-5 minutes on each side, or until cooked through and browned.

<u>To prepare the Mint Cauliflower Rice:</u>

5. Cook the Cauliflower Rice:

In a food processor, pulse the cauliflower florets until they resemble rice in texture.

6. Prepare the Cauliflower Rice:

In a separate skillet over medium heat, heat two tablespoons olive oil.

Sauté the cauliflower rice for 5-7 minutes, or until tender and slightly golden.

7. Season the cauliflower rice as follows:

To the cauliflower rice, add the chopped fresh mint, lemon juice, salt, and pepper.

To combine, stir everything together.

8. Serve:

Serve the carrot meatballs with mint cauliflower rice.

Ingredients:

Regarding the Chicken:

2 skinless, boneless chicken breasts

1 tablespoon olive oil 2 tablespoons mustard

1 teaspoon thyme dried

Paprika, 1/2 teaspoon

1/4 teaspoon red pepper flakes (adjust to desired level of heat)

Add salt and black pepper to taste.

For the Coconut Brussels Sprouts, prepare the following:

2 cups trimmed and halved Brussels sprouts

1 tablespoon unsweetened coconut flakes

1 tablespoon extra-virgin olive oil

Add salt and black pepper to taste.

Instructions:

Regarding the Chicken:

1. Make the marinade:

Combine the Dijon mustard, olive oil, dried thyme, paprika, red pepper flakes, salt, and black pepper in a mixing bowl.

2. Dress the Chicken:

Brush the mustard mixture evenly over the chicken breasts.

3. Marinate:

Allow the chicken to soak up the flavors for at least 15-20 minutes.

4. Prepare the Chicken:

 On medium-high, heat a grill pan or a grill.

Grill the chicken for 6-8 minutes on each side, or until cooked through and charred.

For the Coconut Brussels Sprouts, prepare the following:

5. Roast Brussels sprouts:

Preheat the oven to 400 degrees Fahrenheit (200 degrees Celsius).

Toss the Brussels sprouts with olive oil, salt, and black pepper in a baking dish.

Roast in the oven for 20-25 minutes, or until tender and slightly crispy.

6. Stir in the coconut:

Sprinkle the unsweetened coconut flakes over the Brussels sprouts during the last 5 minutes of roasting and continue roasting until the coconut is toasted.

7. Serve:

Serve with the Coconut Brussels Sprouts and Spicy Mustard Thyme Chicken.

Ingredients:

1 pound large peeled and deveined shrimp

2 tbsp of olive oil

1 finely chopped small onion

2 minced garlic cloves

1 cup halved cherry tomatoes

1 paprika teaspoon

Half teaspoon cumin

Add salt and black pepper to taste.

One lime juice

2 diced ripe avocados

Optional garnish: fresh cilantro

Instructions:

1. Make the Shrimp:

Over medium-high heat, heat 1 tablespoon olive oil in a large skillet

Cook for about 1-2 minutes per side or until the shrimp are pink and opaque. Take the cooked shrimp out of the skillet and set aside.

3. Mix in the tomatoes and spices:

Add the halved cherry tomatoes to the skillet.

Season with paprika, cumin, salt, and black pepper to taste.

Cook for 3-4 minutes, or until the tomatoes soften and begin to release their juices.

4. Mix the shrimp with the lime juice:

Pour the lime juice over the cooked shrimp in the skillet.

 Allow the flavors to meld by cooking for another minute.

5. Include Avocado:

Fold in the diced avocado just before serving. To keep the avocado pieces intact, don't over mix.

6. Decorate and serve:

If desired, garnish with fresh cilantro.

> ➤ Greek Egg Bake

Ingredients:

8 medium eggs

1/2 cup red bell pepper, diced

1/2 cup green bell pepper, diced

1/2 cup red onion, diced

1 pound diced tomatoes

1/2 cup sliced (pitted) Kalamata olives

1 cup spinach leaves, fresh

1/2 cup crumbled feta cheese (use sparingly)

1 tsp. dried oregano

Add salt and black pepper to taste.

Grease the baking dish with olive oil.

Instructions:

1. Preheat the oven to 350°F.

Preheat the oven to 350 degrees Fahrenheit.

2. Lightly grease a baking dish:

To prevent sticking, grease a 9x9-inch baking dish with olive oil.

3. Arrange the Vegetables:

In the bottom of a greased baking dish, arrange the diced red and green bell peppers, red onion, diced tomatoes, Kalamata olives, and fresh spinach in an even layer.

4. Mix in the Feta cheese:

Crumble the feta cheese over the vegetables.

5. Beat the Eggs:

In a separate bowl, whisk the eggs until thoroughly combined.

6. Season and serve:

Season the whisked eggs with oregano, salt, and black pepper to taste.

Evenly distribute the seasoned eggs over the vegetables and feta cheese.

7. Bake:

Place the baking dish in a preheated oven for 25-30 minutes, or until the eggs are set and the top is golden.

8. Serve:

Allow to cool slightly before slicing and serving the Greek Egg Bake.

> ➢ **Tuna Quinoa Salad in Endive Wraps**

Ingredients:

To prepare the Tuna Quinoa Salad:

1 cup cooled cooked quinoa

1 can (5 oz) drained and flaked water-packed tuna

1/2 cup cucumber, diced

1/2 cup red bell pepper, diced

1/4 cup red onion, diced

2 tbsp fresh parsley, chopped

2 tbsp of olive oil

1 teaspoon of lemon juice

Add salt and black pepper to taste.

To make the endive wraps:

1 head Belgian endive (also called chicory)

Garnish with fresh lemon wedges (optional).

Instructions:

To prepare the Tuna Quinoa Salad:

1. Prepare Quinoa:

Cook the quinoa according to package directions, then set it aside to cool to room temperature.

2. Make the Salad:

Combine the cooled quinoa, flaked tuna, diced cucumber, diced red bell pepper, diced red onion, and chopped fresh parsley in a large mixing bowl.

4. Toss and combine:

Dress the tuna quinoa salad with the dressing.

Toss all of the ingredients together gently until evenly coated.

To make the endive wraps:

5. Prepare the endive leaves as follows:

To make small cups, carefully separate the leaves from the head of Belgian endive.

Fill the endive wraps as follows:

Fill the endive cups halfway with the Tuna Quinoa Salad.

7. Serve:

Arrange the endive wraps on a platter to serve.

If desired, garnish with fresh lemon wedges.

> Apple with Cinnamon Almond Butter

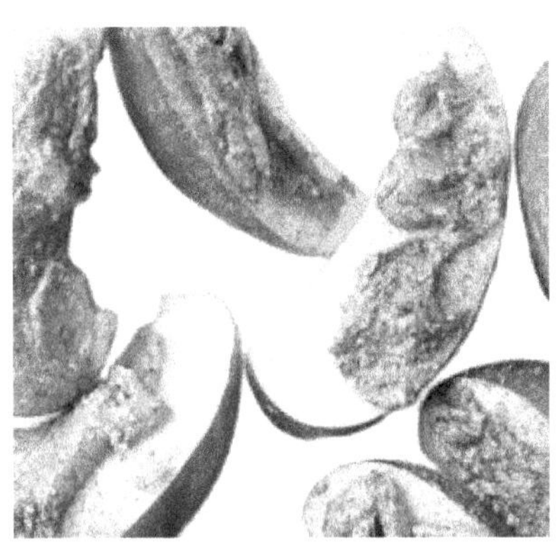

Ingredients:

1 medium apple (your choice of variety)

2 tbsp. unsweetened almond butter

1/2 teaspoon cinnamon powder

Optional: A drizzle of honey or maple syrup (use sparingly or omit for a sugar detox)

Instructions:

1. Make the Apple:

After thoroughly washing the apple, cut it into thin wedges or rounds, removing the core.

2. Construct the Cinnamon Almond Butter:

Combine the almond butter and ground cinnamon in a small bowl.

If you want to add a touch of sweetness, drizzle with honey or maple syrup, but use it sparingly to stay on track with your sugar detox.

3. Dip and Savor:

Dip apple slices in cinnamon almond butter.

Enjoy the delectable blend of flavors and textures.

➢ Cinnamon Sugar Roasted Chickpeas

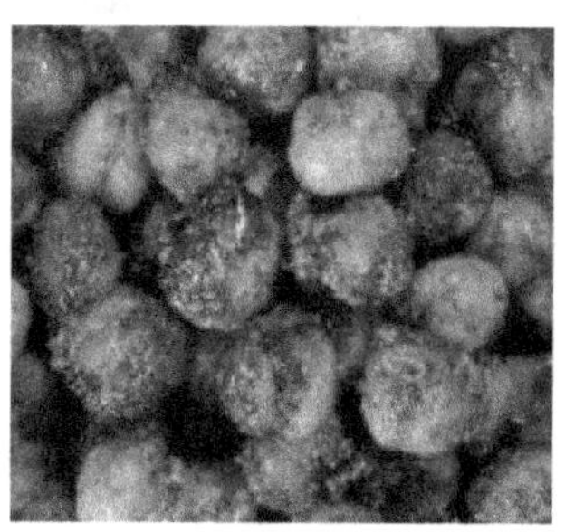

Ingredients:

1 can (15 oz) drained and washed chickpeas (garbanzo beans)

1 tbsp (melted) coconut oil

1 tablespoon cinnamon powder

1/2 teaspoon granulated stevia or monk fruit sweetener (optional sugar-free sweetener)

a quarter teaspoon ground nutmeg

a quarter teaspoon of salt

Instructions:

1. Preheat the oven to 350°F.

Preheat the oven to 375 degrees Fahrenheit.

2. Cook the Chickpeas:

Pat the chickpeas dry with a clean kitchen towel or paper towels after draining and washing them. Excess moisture must be removed for crisper results.

3. Season the chickpeas as follows:

Mix together the dry chickpeas, melted coconut oil, ground cinnamon, granulated stevia or monk fruit sweetener (for a sugar-free alternative), ground nutmeg, and salt in a mixing dish.

Toss the chickpeas in the seasoning until uniformly covered.

4. Roast the Chickpeas:

Line parchment paper on a baking sheet and spread the seasoned chickpeas in a single layer.

5. Bake:

Place the baking pan in the oven and roast the chickpeas for 30-35 minutes, or until golden brown and crispy. Shake the skillet or mix the chickpeas after 15 minutes to ensure balanced cooking.

6. Relax and Have Fun:

Allow to cool before serving the roasted chickpeas.

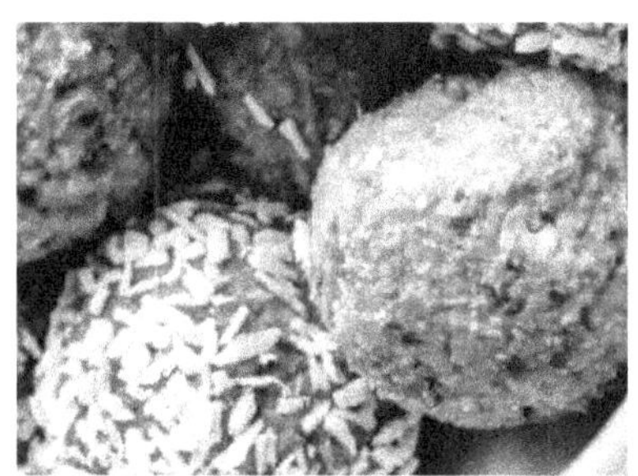

Ingredients:

1 pound rolled oats

1/2 cup carrots, shredded

1/4 cup chopped nuts (walnuts, almonds, or pecans, for example)

1/4 cup shredded unsweetened coconut

1/4 cup unsweetened almond butter

2 tbsp honey or maple syrup (use sparingly or replace with a sugar-free sweetener)

1/2 teaspoon cinnamon powder

a quarter teaspoon ground nutmeg

a quarter teaspoon vanilla extract

Optional: a pinch of salt For extra nourishment, use chia seeds or flaxseeds.

Instructions:

1. Gather the Ingredients:

Use a box grater or food processor to shred the carrots.

If the nuts you've chosen aren't already chopped, cut them into little bits.

2. Combine the Ingredients:

Combine the rolled oats, shredded carrots, chopped almonds, unsweetened shredded coconut, almond butter, honey or maple syrup (or a sugar-free sweetener), cinnamon, nutmeg, vanilla essence, a pinch of salt, and optional chia seeds or flaxseeds in a mixing dish.

3. Thoroughly combine:

In a mixing bowl, combine all the ingredients together. The mixture should be sufficiently sticky to hold together.

4. Create Energy Bites:

Roll little pieces of the mixture into bite-sized energy balls. If the mixture is excessively sticky, moisten your hands to make it easier to handle.

5. Chill:

When the energy bits have firmed up, they are ready to eat.

6. Serve:

Once the energy bites are firm, they are ready to enjoy.

 ➤ Cauliflower Chips

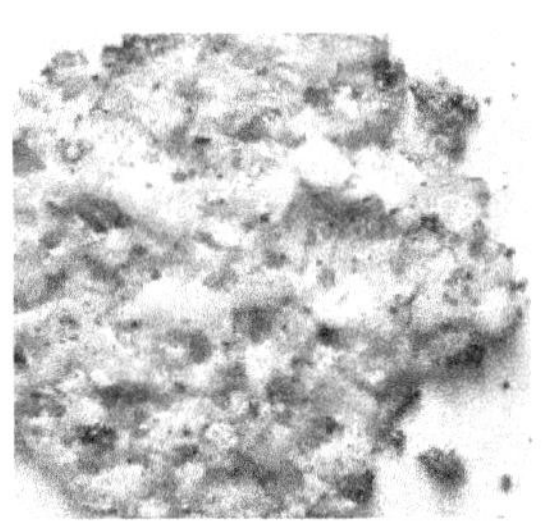

Ingredients:

1 little cauliflower head

2 tbsp of olive oil

1 smoked paprika teaspoon

a half teaspoon garlic powder

A half teaspoon onion powder

Add salt and black pepper to taste.

Instructions:

1. Preheat the oven to 350°F.

Preheat the oven to 400 degrees Fahrenheit.

2. Cook the Cauliflower:

The cauliflower head should be washed and dried.

Remove the cauliflower leaves and chop it into bite-sized florets.

3. Season the cauliflower as follows:

Combine the cauliflower florets, olive oil, smoked paprika, garlic powder, onion powder, salt, and black pepper in a large mixing basin.

4. Coat and Toss:

Toss the cauliflower florets in the seasoning until uniformly covered.

5. Place on a baking sheet:

Place the seasoned cauliflower florets on a parchment-lined baking sheet. To ensure consistent cooking, arrange them in a single layer.

6. Bake:

Bake for 20-25 minutes, or until the cauliflower is cooked and the edges are slightly crispy, in a preheated oven. To ensure even crispiness, turn or flip the florets halfway through cooking time.

7. Allow to cool before serving:

Allow the cauliflower chips to cool for a few minutes before serving.

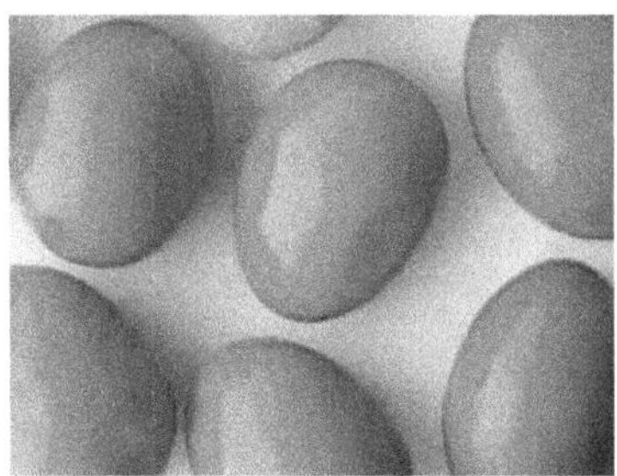

Ingredients:

Six huge eggs

1 cup distilled white vinegar

1 cup of water

1 tablespoon sugar-free granulated stevia or monk fruit sweetener

1 teaspoon sea salt

1/2 teaspoon ground black pepper

1 tablespoon mustard seeds

1/2 teaspoon coriander seeds, whole

1/2 teaspoon dried red pepper flakes (adjust to desired amount of heat)

2-3 garlic cloves, peeled and crushed

2-3 fresh dill sprigs (optional, for extra taste)

Instructions:

1. Cook the eggs hard:

Fill a pot halfway with water and add the eggs.

Bring the water to a boil, then reduce to a low heat and cook for 9-12 minutes.

When the eggs are hard-boiled, place them in an ice bath to chill. This makes peeling simpler.

2. Remove the shells from the eggs:

Peel the eggs and set them aside when they have cooled.

3. Construct the Pickling Liquid:

To make a sugar-free version, mix the white vinegar, water, granulated stevia or monk fruit sweetener, salt, black peppercorns, mustard seeds, entire coriander seeds, dried red pepper flakes, and crushed garlic cloves in a skillet.

4. Warm up the Pickling Liquid:

Bring the pickling liquid to a boil, then lower to a low heat and allow the flavors to mingle for about 5 minutes.

5. Pickled Eggs:

Fill a clean, disinfected glass jar or container halfway with peeled eggs. Fresh dill sprigs can be added for additional taste if desired.

6. Pour in the Pickling Liquid:

Make sure the eggs in the jar are completely covered before carefully pouring the hot pickling liquid over them. To get rid of any air bubbles, you might need to give the jar a little tap.

7. Chill Out and Store:

Allow the liquid and pickled eggs to come to room temperature.

Before consuming, seal the jar or container and place it in the refrigerator for at least 24 hours. They will get more flavorful the longer you keep them in the fridge.

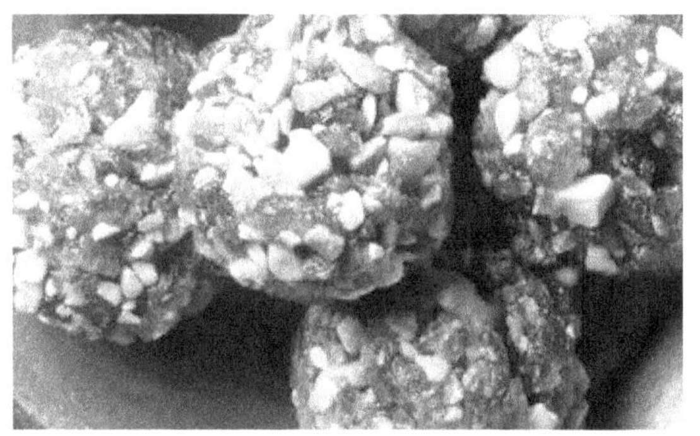

Ingredients:

10 pitted Medjool dates

1/2 cup shelled unsalted pistachios

1 teaspoon cumin powder

1 tablespoon smoked paprika

1/4 teaspoon coriander powder

1/4 teaspoon ground black pepper

Pinch of salt (OPTIONAL)

1 lemon's zest

1 tablespoon extra-virgin olive oil

Instructions:

1. Set the dates:

Remove the pits from the dates if they haven't already been pitted.

2. Pistachios, toasted:

Toast the pistachios in a dry skillet over medium heat for 2-3 minutes, or until fragrant. To avoid burning, make sure to stir them frequently. Allow them to cool after they have been toasted.

3. Combine the following ingredients:

Combine the pitted dates, toasted pistachios, ground cumin, smoked paprika, ground coriander, black pepper, and a pinch of salt (if using) in a food processor.

4. Combine by pulsing:

Pulse the ingredients until a sticky, coarse mixture forms. For texture, use small pistachio chunks.

5. Stir in the lemon zest and olive oil:

To the mixture, add the lemon zest and olive oil. Continue the process repeatedly until everything is well combined.

6. Form into Bites:

Scoop small amounts of the mixture and roll into bite-sized balls.

7. Refrigerate and serve:

Refrigerate the savory date and pistachio bites for at least 30 minutes to firm up.

Optional garnishes:

Before chilling, roll the bites in additional crushed pistachios or a sprinkle of smoked paprika for a finishing touch.

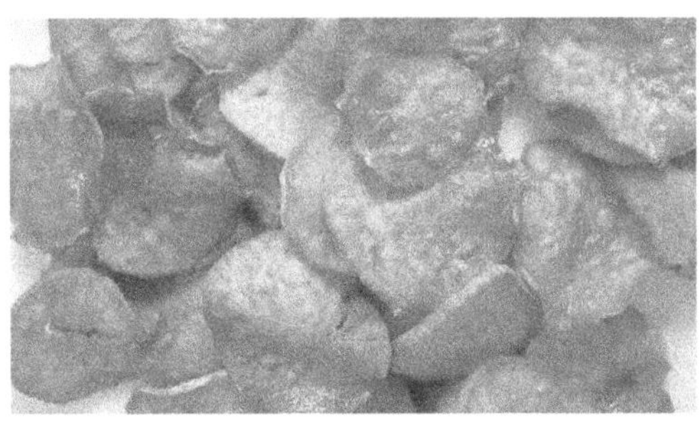

Ingredients:

2 medium washed and peeled sweet potatoes

2 tbsp of olive oil

1 smoked paprika teaspoon

a half teaspoon garlic powder

a half teaspoon onion powder

1/4 teaspoon cayenne pepper (to taste)

Season with salt to taste

Instructions:

1. Preheat the oven to 350°F.

Preheat the oven to 375 degrees Fahrenheit.

2. Cut the sweet potatoes into slices:

Thinly slice the sweet potatoes into rounds with a mandoline slicer or a sharp knife. For even baking, aim for uniform thickness.

3. Make the seasonings:

Combine the olive oil, smoked paprika, garlic powder, onion powder, cayenne pepper, and salt in a small mixing bowl.

4. Gently toss the sweet potatoes:

In a large mixing bowl, combine the sweet potato slices. Toss the slices in the seasoned olive oil mixture until they are evenly coated.

5. Arrange on baking sheets as follows:

Arrange the sweet potato slices on baking sheets lined with parchment paper in a single layer. To ensure even baking, make sure they are not overlapping.

6. Bake:

Bake for 15-20 minutes, flipping halfway through, or until the sweet potato chips are crisp and golden brown around the edges.

7. Allow to cool before serving:

Allow the sweet potato chips to cool on a cooling rack. As they cool, they will continue to crisp up.

8. Seasonings are optional.

If desired, season the chips with additional salt or your favorite spice blend while they are still warm.

> **Super Seed Snack Bars**

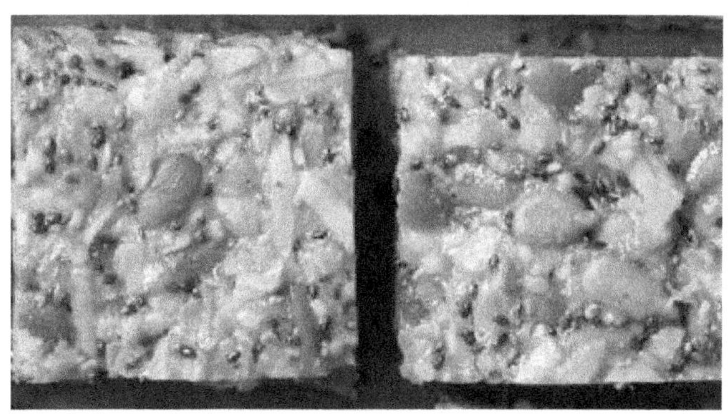

Ingredients:

1 cup mixed seeds (chia, flax, pumpkin, and sunflower seeds)

1 cup chopped nuts (almonds, walnuts, or a combination)

1/2 cup shredded unsweetened coconut

1/2 cup nut butter (almond butter, peanut butter, or your preferred nut butter)

1/3 cup sugar-free sweetener (such as stevia or monk fruit)

1/4 cup melted coconut oil

A tsp. vanilla extract

Pinch of salt

Optional add in:

Cacao nibs or sugar-free chocolate chips, 1/4 cup

1/4 cup dried berries (unsweetened cranberries or blueberries preferred)

Instructions:

1. Prepare the Nuts and Seeds:

Combine the mixed seeds, chopped nuts, and unsweetened shredded coconut in a large mixing bowl.

2. Construct the Binding Mixture:

Use a separate microwave-safe bowl to melt the coconut oil. Combine the nut butter, sugar-free sweetener, vanilla extract, and a pinch of salt in a mixing bowl. Mix until everything is well combined.

3. Mix Wet and Dry Ingredients:

Pour the wet ingredients over the seeds and nuts.

Continue to mix until all of the ingredients are evenly coated.

4. Add the following optional ingredients:

To add flavor, fold in cacao nibs or sugar-free chocolate chips and dried berries.

5. Place in a pan:

Using parchment paper, line a square baking dish. Transfer the mixture to the dish and firmly press it down to form an even layer.

6. Chill:

Refrigerate the dish for at least 2-3 hours, or until the mixture has hardened.

7. Cut the bars:

Remove from the refrigerator once chilled and firm, and cut into bars.

8. Store:

Refrigerate the bars in an airtight container to keep them fresh. They can also be individually wrapped for easy grab-and-go.

> strawberry oat streusel balls

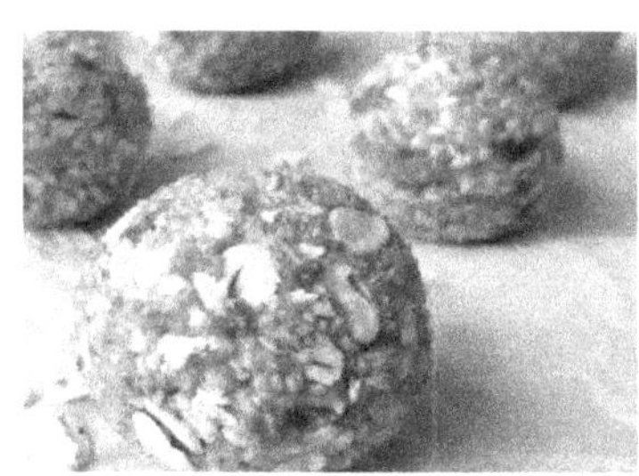

Ingredients:

Filling with strawberries:

1 cup hulled and diced fresh strawberries

1 teaspoon chia seeds

1 tbsp sugar-free sweetener (such as stevia or monk fruit sweetener)

1 tsp. lemon juice

To make the Oat Streusel:

1 pound rolled oats

1 pound almond flour

1/4 cup melted coconut oil

2 tbsp sugar-free sweetener (such as stevia or monk fruit sweetener)

a half teaspoon of vanilla extract

1 teaspoon salt

Instructions:

1. Begin by making the strawberry filling:

Combine the chopped strawberries, chia seeds, sugar-free sweetener, and lemon juice in a small saucepan.

Cook, stirring regularly, over medium heat until the strawberries break down and the liquid thickens to a jam-like consistency.

Remove from the heat and set aside to cool.

2. Prepare the Oat Streusel

Combine rolled oats, almond flour, melted coconut oil, sugar-free sweetener, vanilla extract, and a sprinkle of salt in a large mixing basin.

Mix the ingredients until they form a crumbly streusel.

3. Put the Balls Together:

Press a tiny amount of the oat streusel mixture flat in the palm of your hand.

Spoon a little quantity of strawberry filling into the middle and wrap the streusel mixture around the filling to make a ball. Repeat until all of the mixture has been used.

4. Chill:

Place the strawberry oat streusel balls on a dish or tray and place in the refrigerator to harden up for at least 30 minutes.

5. Serve:

The strawberry oat streusel balls are ready to serve once cooled.

CONCLUSION

Staying Sugar-Free Beyond 30 Days

Tips for Maintaining a Low-Sugar Lifestyle

Educate Yourself: Begin by learning where hidden sugars may be found. Learn to read product labels and recognize sugar alternatives such as sucrose, high fructose corn syrup, and agave nectar.

Plan Balanced Meals: Create meals with a variety of macronutrients, such as lean proteins, healthy fats, and complex carbs. This aids in blood sugar stabilization and lowers cravings for sugary foods.

Select entire Foods: Choose entire, unprocessed foods such as fruits and vegetables, lean meats, and whole grains. These meals include necessary nutrients while avoiding the additional sugars present in many processed foods.

Stay hydrated: Drink lots of water throughout the day to stay hydrated. Sometimes the body misinterprets thirst for hunger, resulting in unneeded sugary munching.

Snack wisely: Snack wisely by selecting nutrient-dense foods such as raw almonds, seeds, or veggies with hummus. These choices give long-lasting energy without causing blood sugar increases like sugary foods.

Mindful Eating: Watch your portion amounts and relish each meal. Eating thoughtfully can help prevent overeating and lessen the probability of habitually reaching for sweet foods.

Gradual reduction: Instead of stopping sugar all at once, consider gradually lowering your intake. This method helps the taste receptors and the body to adjust more easily.

Artificial Sweeteners: Exercise caution while using artificial sweeteners. While they appear to be a sugar-free option, certain researches indicate that they might nevertheless cause cravings for sweet foods. In moderation, use natural sweeteners such as stevia or monk fruit.

Meal Planning and Preparation: **Plan** and prepare meals ahead of time to avoid depending on convenience items containing hidden sugars. Having healthy, homemade options on hand might help minimize impulsive, sugary decisions.

Manage Stress: Emotional eating and sugar cravings can be caused by chronic stress. Incorporate stress-reduction practices into your routine, such as meditation, yoga, or deep breathing exercises.

Get Enough Sleep: **Sleep** deprivation might interfere with hunger hormones and boost cravings for high-calorie, sugary meals. To enhance general health and well-being, aim for 7-9 hours of excellent sleep every night.

Celebrate Successes: **Recognize** and celebrate accomplishments along the road. Recognizing progress, whether it's successfully rejecting a sweet temptation or reaching a goal, can help promote healthy habits.

Remember that transitioning to a low-sugar lifestyle is a gradual process, and everyone's path is different. Adapt these suggestions to your personal preferences and lifestyle while aiming for long-term, sustainable improvements.

How to Handle Sugar Cravings

Sugar cravings can be difficult to manage, but with conscious tactics, they can be effectively navigated. Here are some suggestions for dealing with sugar cravings when on a sugar detox plan:

Keep Hydrated:

Dehydration is sometimes confused with hunger or sugar cravings. When a hunger strikes, drink a glass of water and wait a few minutes to see whether the yearning goes away.

Select Whole Fruits:

When sugar cravings come, go for entire fruits. They include natural sweetness as well as fiber, which can help maintain blood sugar levels and control cravings.

Include Protein in Your Diet:

Protein-rich meals can help you feel fuller for longer and minimize your chances of desiring sweets. Include lean meats, fish, eggs, dairy, and plant-based proteins into your diet.

Satiety-Inducing healthy Fats:

Add healthy fats in your diet, such as avocados, nuts, seeds, and olive oil. Fats increase satiety, lowering the desire to munch on sweet foods.

Plan Healthy Snacks:

Prepare balanced snacks that contain protein, healthy fats, and fiber. Satisfying alternatives include Greek yogurt with berries, nut butter on apple slices, and vegetables with hummus.

Mindful Eating Techniques:

Savor each bite and pay attention to the flavors and sensations of your food to practice mindful eating. This can increase the enjoyment you experience from your meals while decreasing your urge for sweet indulgences.

Determine Triggers:

Recognize events or feelings that cause you to crave sweets. Cravings can be triggered by stress, boredom, or certain settings. Once these triggers have been recognized, concentrate on developing healthy coping methods for them.

Start Moving:

When you have a hunger, engage in some physical exercise. Exercise can help relieve stress and raise mood, making cravings less likely to take hold.

Rest Well:

Ensure you receive enough and good quality sleeps. Sleep deprivation can alter hunger hormones and boost appetites for sweet meals. Maintain a regular sleep schedule for optimal overall health.

Look for sugar-free alternatives to your favorite sweets. Sugar-free gum, herbal teas, or snacks sweetened with natural alternatives such as stevia or monk fruit, for example, can give a hint of sweetness without the use of additional sugars.

Divert Your Attention:

When a hunger strikes, do something you like to divert yourself. Going for a stroll, reading a book, or indulging in a pastime will help you divert your attention away from the urge.

Not Perfection, but Progress:

Recognize that occasional cravings are normal. Instead of perceiving them as failures, consider them chances to strengthen your dedication to a low-sugar lifestyle. Perfection is less essential than progress.

Discuss your sugar detox with friends, family, or a support group. Sharing your experiences and receiving support might help to make the process less stressful.

Remember that getting free from sugar cravings takes time, and each positive choice you make helps to your overall well-being. As you attempt to maintain a low-sugar lifestyle, consistency and patience are essential.

The Long-Term Benefits of a Sugar Detox

A sugar detox plan can provide various long-term benefits for women, improving both physical health and overall well-being. Here are some of the long-term benefits:

Weight Control:

A sugar detox is frequently associated with weight reduction and improved weight control. Reduced added sugar consumption can help manage hunger, lower overall calorie intake, and promote a better body composition.

Blood sugar levels that are stable:

Individuals can achieve more stable blood sugar levels by avoiding or limiting their intake of processed sweets. This can help maintain energy levels, boost mood, and lower the risk of developing insulin resistance and type 2 diabetes.

Heart Health Improvement:

Sugar reduction has been linked to better heart health. A sugar detox can result in lower triglyceride levels, blood pressure, and risk factors for cardiovascular disease.

Improved Mental Clarity:

Excess sugar consumption has been related to cognitive problems as well as an increased risk of neurodegenerative illnesses. A sugar detox may enhance brain clarity, attention, and reduce the risk of illnesses such as Alzheimer's disease.

Inflammation is reduced:

Excess sugar consumption can contribute to chronic inflammation, which has been related to a variety of health problems such as arthritis, heart disease, and some malignancies. A sugar detox may assist to decrease inflammation, resulting in better overall health.

Improved Skin Health:

Sugar consumption should be reduced to improve skin health. High sugar consumption has been linked to skin problems such as acne and premature aging. A sugar detox may result in healthier skin and a more youthful appearance.

Hormone Balance:

Sugar intake has the potential to disrupt hormone balance, notably insulin and cortisol. A sugar detox may help to enhance reproductive health, mood, and minimize PMS symptoms by balancing these hormones.

Improved Digestive Health:

Processed sugars can upset the balance of gut flora and cause digestive problems. A sugar detox, paired with a fiber- and whole-food-rich diet, can help to sustain a healthy gut micro biota and enhance digestive function.

Chronic Disease Risk is Reduced:

Sugar consumption is linked to a lower risk of chronic illnesses such as type 2 diabetes, some malignancies, and metabolic syndrome. Adherence to a low-sugar lifestyle over time may contribute to a decreased overall risk of these illnesses.

Increased Vitality and Energy:

Stable blood sugar levels and enhanced metabolic function as a result of a sugar detox can lead to increased energy and vitality. This can improve everyday activities, athletic performance, and general quality of life.

Developing Healthy Habits:

Adopting healthy eating habits is typically part of a sugar detox. Individuals may develop a higher appreciation for nutrient-dense meals, mindful eating, and overall healthier lifestyle choices over time.

Positive Emotional Well-Being Impact:

Blood sugar levels that are steady contribute to mood stability. Excess sugar consumption can reduce mood fluctuations, anxiety, and irritation, resulting to improved emotional well-being.

In conclusion, a sugar detox plan can provide several long-term advantages, including improved physical health, emotional well-being, and the prevention of chronic illnesses. The favorable changes that occur during a sugar detox can pave the way for a long-term, healthier lifestyle.

This comprehensive cookbook and 30-day plan will empower you as a woman to take control of your health, kick sugar cravings to the curb, and achieve that weight loss goals while enjoying delicious, nutritious meals, snacks and smoothies.

"Thank you for choosing the Sugar Detox Cookbook! Your dedication to health is inspiring. "Enjoy the tasty journey to wellness

Enjoying the recipes of this book, kindly leave a review!!!

Thank you

www.ingramcontent.com/pod-product-compliance
Lightning Source LLC
Chambersburg PA
CBHW070926260726
48661CB00003B/842